Essentials of Physical Education

Essentials of Physical Education

Aria Kramer

SYRAWOOD
PUBLISHING HOUSE
New York

Published by Syrawood Publishing House,
750 Third Avenue, 9th Floor,
New York, NY 10017, USA
www.syrawoodpublishinghouse.com

Essentials of Physical Education
Aria Kramer

International Standard Book Number: 978-1-68286-822-5 (Hardback)

Cataloging-in-Publication Data

Essentials of physical education / Aria Kramer.
p. cm.
Includes bibliographical references and index.
ISBN 978-1-68286-822-5
1. Physical education and training. 2. Sports. I. Kramer, Aria.

GV341 .E77 2019
613.7--dc23

Printed in China.

TABLE OF CONTENTS

PREFACE

Physical education is an educational discipline related to the maintenance of human health through physical exercises. Such education emphasizes on psychomotor learning and is imparted to children between primary and secondary education. Physical education is important for the overall health and well-being of students. It encompasses a wide variety of physical activities such as hiking, bowling, Frisbee, regular sports and yoga as well as self-defense and martial arts. The curriculum is generally designed to provide exposure to aquatics, gymnastics, dance, rhythms, team sports, etc. Trainers and educators can use the technologies of heart rate monitors and pedometers to measure and set goals for fitness. This book unfolds the innovative aspects of physical education, which will be crucial for the holistic understanding of the subject matter. Different approaches, evaluations, methodologies and advanced studies in this discipline have been included herein. This book will serve as a reference to a broad spectrum of readers.

A detailed account of the significant topics covered in this book is provided below:

Chapter 1- Physical education is an educational course for students at primary and secondary level of education related to the promotion of health of the human body through physical exercise and psychomotor learning. This is an introductory chapter, which will introduce briefly all the significant aspects of physical education, physical exercise, physical fitness and physical literacy.

Chapter 2- Gymnastics is a sport or a set of exercises that involves coordination, physical agility, strength, flexibility and endurance. All the major muscle groups such as those of the arms, legs, back, shoulders, chest and the abdomen are stimulated in gymnastics. The topics elaborated in this chapter include acrobatic gymnastics, artistic gymnastics, rhythmic gymnastics, floor gymnastics, etc.

Chapter 3- Aerobics is a form of physical activity, which combines strength training with rhythmic aerobic exercise with the objective of augmenting flexibility, cardio-vascular fitness and muscular strength. The diverse forms of aerobic exercise, such as indoor aerobic exercises and outdoor aerobic exercises have been thoroughly discussed in this chapter.

Chapter 4- Swimming is a recreational activity, an exercise or a sport involved with the self-propulsion of an individual in water using his/her arms and legs. The aim of this chapter is to explore the principal topics of resistance swimming and swimming stroke with respect to physical education. It explores the different types of swimming strokes, such as front crawl, butterfly stroke, breaststroke, backstroke, sidestroke, etc.

Chapter 5- Weight training is a form of strength training that involves the development of strength and size of the skeletal muscles, using dumbbells, weighted bars and weight stacks. A weight training regime is a significant aspect of physical education. This chapter discusses in detail the relevant weight training exercises, such as squats, leg presses, biceps training, triceps training, etc.

Chapter 6- Regular exercise and sports maintain the overall health and wellness of the body and enhances physical fitness. Different sports help in maintaining physical fitness. Extensive importance is laid on sports, such as tennis, basketball, football, etc. in physical education, which have been thoroughly discussed in this chapter.

It gives me an immense pleasure to thank our entire team for their efforts. Finally in the end, I would like to thank my family and colleagues who have been a great source of inspiration and support.

Aria Kramer

Chapter 1

An Introduction to Physical Education

Physical education is an educational course for students at primary and secondary level of education related to the promotion of health of the human body through physical exercise and psychomotor learning. This is an introductory chapter, which will introduce briefly all the significant aspects of physical education, physical exercise, physical fitness and physical literacy.

Physical education is a course taught in school that focuses on developing physical fitness and the ability to perform and enjoy day-to-day physical activities with ease. Kids also develop skills necessary to participate in a wide range of activities, such as soccer, basketball, or swimming. Regular physical education classes prepare kids to be physically and mentally active, fit, and healthy into adulthood. An effective physical education program should include engaging lessons, trained P.E. teachers, adequate instructional periods, and student evaluation.

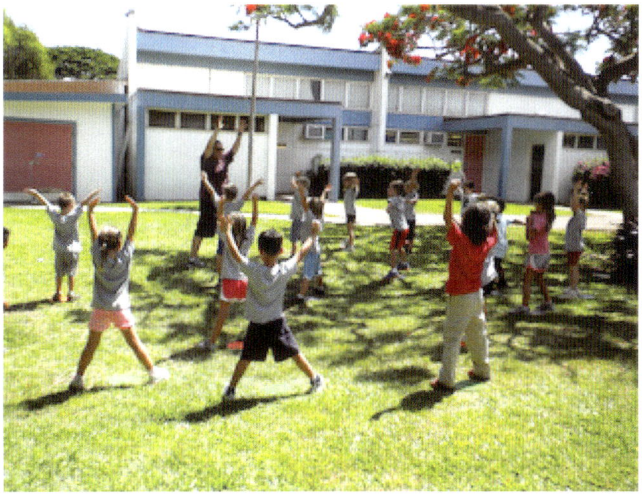

Physical Education Curriculum

Physical education helps students develop physical skills and confidence. For example, elementary and middle school curriculum includes activities that help kids obtain and improve skills, such as running, catching, throwing, and striking, applicable to sports such as baseball, volleyball, or karate. Balancing skills could be applied to dance or gymnastics.

High school curriculum should focus on lifetime sports skills like tennis or aerobic dance, with a secondary emphasis on team sports.

Physical education develops fitness and fosters the desire for lifelong participation in physical activity. high school curriculum prepares students to become highly proficient in one or more sport and/or fitness activity of their choice.

Physical education classes teach the health benefits of regular exercise and healthy food choices along with the risks of inactivity and poor diet. Students of all ages might be asked to dedicate themselves to making a few small improvements in diet and exercise for a period of six weeks. They would be expected to journal about how they feel during the process and reflect on how these changes affect performance and mood.

Physical education also helps students develop social skills. For example, team sports help them learn to respect others, contribute to a team goal, and socialize as a productive member of a team.

To understand what physical education, we must understand physical fitness which it intends to promote. Physical fitness is comprised of the following:

Cardiovascular fitness - This is the ability of your heart and lungs to deliver the oxygen your body needs for its daily tasks. This is the fitness component that is addressed by such aerobic activities as brisk walking, jogging, running, dancing and swimming.

Strength - This is the amount physical power that a muscle or group of muscles can use against a weight or resistance. This is addressed by such activities as weight lifting and body weight training.

Endurance -This is the ability of a muscle or group of muscles to repeat movements or hold a position over a certain period of time. Long-distance running is an activity that helps to develop endurance.

Flexibility - This refers to the body's range of movement. Pilates, yoga and gymnastics help promote this particular fitness component.

Body composition - This refers to the ratio of the body's fat component vs. its lean mass. Exercises that address cardiovascular fitness, strength, endurance and flexibility also promote the reduction of fat and the build-up of muscle.

Builds Self-Confidence

The participation in physical education in high school provides a positive influence on a student's personality, character and self-esteem. In addition, the team-building process enhances communication skills, and the skills required to get along and cooperate with students of varying ethnic backgrounds and personalities.

Develops Motor Skills

Physical education in high school is essential to the development of motor skills and the enhancement of reflexes. Hand-eye coordination is improved, as well as good body movements, which helps in the development of a healthy body posture.

Health and Nutrition

Physical education teaches students the importance of physical health. High school is an age where students misinterpret the meaning of "overweight" and eating disorders prevail. Physical health and education informs students on sound eating practices and the essential guidelines for nutrition.

Relieves Stress

High school students have substantial amounts of stress due to curriculum, homework, families and peer pressures. Involvement in sports, recreational activities or other forms of physical fitness offer a method of stress relief.

Trends

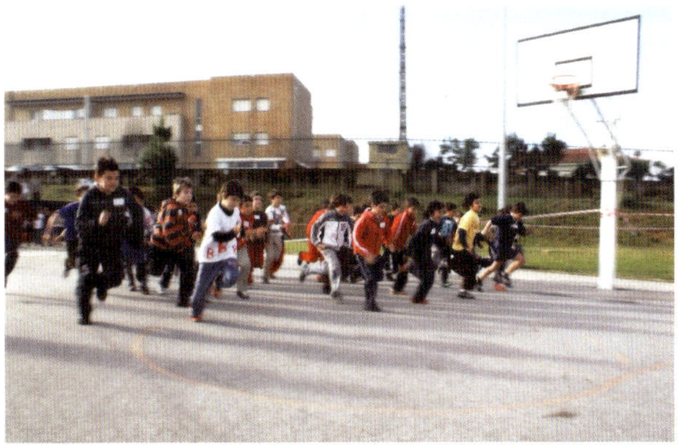

Young Portuguese children participating in a school race

Physical education trends have developed recently to incorporate a greater variety of activities besides typical sports. Introducing students to activities like bowling, walking/hiking, or frisbee at an early age can help them develop good activity habits that will continue into adulthood.

Some teachers have begun to incorporate stress-reduction techniques such as yoga, deep breathing and tai chi. Tai chi, an ancient martial arts form focused on slow meditative movements, is a relaxation activity with many benefits. Studies have shown that it enhances muscular strength and endurance, as well as cardiovascular endurance. It also provides psychological benefits such as improving general mental health, concentration, awareness and positive mood. It can be taught to any age student with little or no equipment, making it ideal for mixed ability and age classes. Tai chi can easily be incorporated into a holistic learning body and mind unit.

Teaching non-traditional sports may also provide motivation for students to increase their activity, and can help them learn about different cultures. For example, while learning about lacrosse in the Southwestern United States, students might also learn about the Native American cultures of the Northeastern United States and Eastern Canada, where the sport originated. Teaching non-traditional (or non-native) sports provides an opportunity to integrate academic concepts from other subjects as well, which may now be required of many PE teachers.

PE is very important to students' health and overall well-being. The Centers for Disease Control and Prevention stated that over the past three years obesity in children (ages 2–5) and adolescents (ages 12–19) has doubled because of diet and lack of activity. Since the 1970s the number of children who are obese has tripled.

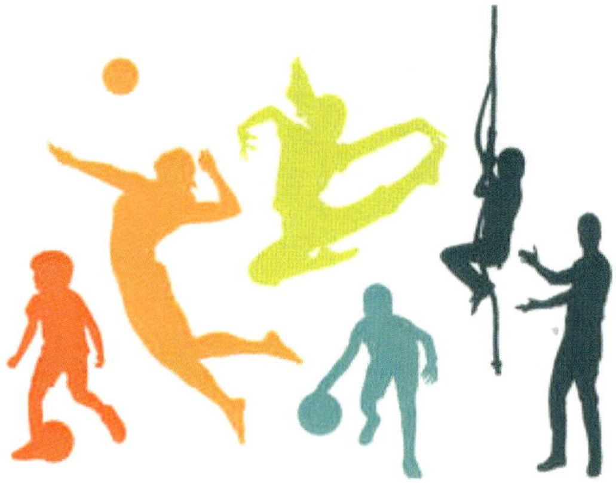

SHAPE America's National Standards & Grade-Level Outcomes for K-12 Physical Education define what a student should know and be able to do as result of an effective physical education program.

Another trend is the incorporation of health and nutrition into the physical education curriculum. The Child Nutrition and WIC Reauthorization Act of 2004 required that all school districts with a federally-funded school meal program develop wellness policies that address nutrition and physical activity. While teaching students sports and movement skills, PE teachers are now incorporating short health and nutrition lessons into the curriculum. This is more prevalent at the elementary school level, where students do not have a specific Health class. Recently most elementary schools have specific health classes for students as well as physical education class. Due to the recent outbreaks of diseases such as swine flu, school districts are making it mandatory for students to learn about practicing good hygiene along with other health topics.

Today many states require Physical Education teachers to be certified to teach Health courses. Many colleges and universities offer both Physical Education and Health as one certification. This push towards health education is beginning at the intermediate level, including lessons on bullying, self-esteem and stress and anger management.

Research has shown that there is a positive correlation between brain development and exercising.

Incorporating local indigenous knowledge into physical education can lead to many meaningful experiences and a way of learning about other cultures. For example, by incorporating traditional knowledge from varying indigenous groups from across Canada, students can be exposed to many concepts such as holistic learning and the medicine wheel. A unit could be focused on connecting to a place or feeling while outdoors, participating in traditional games, or outdoor environmental education. These types of lesson can easily be integrated into other parts of the curriculum and give Aboriginal students a chance to incorporate their culture in the local school community.

Studies have been done in how physical education can help improve academic achievement. In a 2007 article, researchers found a profound gain in English Arts standardized testing test scores among students who had 56 hours of physical education in a year, compared to those who had 28 hours of physical education a year.

In Brazil, the physical education curriculum is designed to allow school pupils a full range of modern opportunities, including sports. Martial arts classes, like wrestling in the United States, and Pencak Silat in France, Indonesia, and Malaysia, teach children self-defense and to feel good about themselves. The physical education curriculum is designed to allow students to experience at least a minimum exposure to the following categories of activities: aquatics, conditioning activities, gymnastics, individual/dual sports, team sports, rhythms, and dance.

In these areas, a planned sequence of learning experiences is designed to support a progression of student development. This allows kids through 6th grade to be introduced to sports, fitness, and teamwork in order to be better prepared for the middle and high school age. In 1975, the United States House of Representatives voted to require school physical education classes include both genders. Some high school and some middle school PE classes are single-sex.

Technology use in Physical Education

New technology in education is playing a big role in classes. One of the most affordable and effective tools is a simple video recorder. With this, students can see the mistakes they're making in things such as a throwing motion or swinging form. Studies show that students find this more effective than having someone try to explain what they are doing wrong, and then trying to correct it. Educators may use technologies such as pedometers and heart rate monitors to make step and heart rate goals for students.

Other technologies that can be used in a Physical Education setting include video projectors, GPS and games and gaming systems such as Kinect, Wii Fit and *Dance Dance Revolution*. Projectors can show students proper form or how to play certain games. GPS systems can be used to get students active in an outdoor setting, and active exergames can be used by teachers to show students a good way to stay fit in and out of the classroom setting.

Another type of technology that is commonly used in Physical Education is the pedometer. This does not necessarily track how far a person is going, but lets them know the number of steps they are taking.

Adapted Physical Education

Adapted physical education (APE) is physical education that is individualized and specially designed to address the needs of students with disabilities who require adaptations or modifications to be physically active, and participate safely.

Federal law mandates that physical education be provided to students with disabilities and defines Physical Education as the development of:

- physical and motor skills
- fundamental motor skills and patterns (throwing, catching, walking, running, etc)
- skills in aquatics, dance, and individual and group games and sports (including intramural and lifetime sports)

The Individuals with Disabilities Education Act (1990) uses the term disability as a diagnostic category that qualifies students for special services. These categories include:

- Autism
- Deaf – Blindness

- Deafness
- Hearing impairment
- Intellectual disability
- Multiple disabilities
- Orthopedic impairment
- Other health impairment
- Serious emotional disturbance
- Specific learning disability
- Speech or language impairment
- Traumatic brain injury
- Visual impairment including blindness

The services provided by an APE teacher include:

- Planning services
- Assessment of Individuals /Ecosystems
- Prescription/Placement: The IEP
- Teaching/Counseling/Coaching
- Evaluation of Services
- Coordination of Resources and Consulting
- Advocacy

The APE teacher is a direct service provider, not a related service provider, because physical education for children with disabilities is a federally mandated component of special education services. This means that physical education needs to be provided to the student with a disability as part of the special education services that child and family receive. This is contrasted with physical therapy and occupational therapy, which are related services. These therapies are provided to the child with disabilities only if he/she needs them to benefit from instruction.

Teaching for Specific Disabilities

Intellectual Disabilities

There are a number of general modifications that can be applied in a physical education environment for students with intellectual disabilities.

The first set of modifications deal with communication. When instructing students use shorter sentences, use gestures or demonstrations as supplement to verbal cues, repeat directions and have students repeat directions back to you, provide praise often, and give more feedback.

The next set of modifications deal with practice. Give students extra practice trials, build in more time for a student to master skills, make sure activities are perceived as fun, promote active participation, shorten activities to reduce problems with attention span, and allow choices in what activity will be done, when it will be done, where it will take place, and with whom the child will participate in the activity with. One method to structure activities is known as level teaching. To accommodate for students with varying levels of intellectual disabilities a game will be designed with different levels. For example, if the specific sport is volleyball the instructor will set up 3 courts with different modifications at each court to accommodate for these varying levels of disability. Court 1 may have a set of cones designating opposing sides while Court 3 has a net set in place. Different rules may be applied to different courts as well, allowing every student to be challenged in a constructive way.

The third set of modifications deal with curriculum. Adjust the general education curriculum to meet the needs of a student. For example, reduce the number of objectives that need to be mastered. If a student is severely delayed, an entirely new curriculum may need to be made. Activities may also need to provide early success which will encourage adherence.

The final set of modifications deal with the environment. It should be structured and visually appealing. It is essential to reduce playing areas in order to eliminate distractions. Plan to structure the environment in a way that will allow you to deal with behavioral problems.

Learning Disabilities

1 in 5 students with learning disabilities will also have motor impairments. There are a number of ways to accommodate these students.

Reduce class size: This allows teacher extra one on one time with students. Often a class of 20-30 students proves to be more effective than double or triple that in general physical education classes.

Use peer tutors: Peers can be rained in how to provide specific skill feedback as well as modify activities so the student has higher success. This can be effective when class size cannot be reduced.

Offer learning strategies: Both teachers and peer tutors can provide strategies to help disorganized learners focus. This includes provided picture cues, video cues, and additional cues such as footprints on the floor to help a student understand what and how to perform an activity.

Provide structured practice: Allow the student to get many practice opportunities. This will help them learn how to listen to and observe visual feedback for performance.

Identify success: Reframe success for students in a way that does not focus on the end result. For example, using correct form in shooting should be a measure of success rather than making the basket.

Use a variety of senses when giving instructions: Some students do better listening to instruction while others do better watching a demonstration. Others may do best when physically guided into the pattern. By incorporating many types of learning styles, students will be more likely to succeed.

ADHD

Students with attention-deficit/hyperactivity disorder may experience motor learning delays. Many strategies are available to minimize learning delays in students with ADHD.

Positive feedback: There is a relationship between positive feedback given by a physical education teacher and students applying corrective feedback.

Task sheets: A task sheet provides a progression of activities to be completed by the students and requires them to record their results. Task sheets can be turned in at the end of class. This allows students to assess their performance while acknowledging their need to improve their skills.

Token economy or point system: This is a structured agreement between the student and teacher in which the student earns rewards by meeting a minimum expectation. At the end of class both the student and teacher initial the points earned. At the end of the month, the student may earn a reward of his or her choice provided by the teacher.

Autism Spectrum Disorder

Various strategies exist to allow students with autism to be successfully included in a physical education setting.

Preparing for inclusion: It is essential to know the students needs, abilities, and preferences. It is also important to prepare the student. The physical education environment may be anxiety inducing for them. Because of this, educators can slowly introduce the student to the environment. They may also preview the class using visual organizers to describe the setting the student will be a part of. They may also make visual schedules prior to class. It is also important to prepare the peers by teaching them what autism is and behaviors associated with it.

Instructing the student: There are a variety of methods for instructing students with autism. The first, environmental prompts. This involves the intentional use of equipment to encourage specific behaviors. The next is verbal prompts. This includes avoiding negative sentences. For example, instruction such as "step with your right leg" as opposed to "don't step with your left leg". Verbal prompts also include keeping phrases literal as well as provided concise instruction. It is also important to be consistent with language use. Peer tutors may also provide a lot of benefits for students in the physical education setting.

Deafness

Being deaf or hard of hearing typically has little impact on the development of motor skills, fitness levels, and participation in sports. However, it is still important to accommodate students who are deaf or hard of hearing in the physical education setting.

Communicate using his or her preferred means of communication. When giving verbal instructions, make sure the student can see the instructors face clearly. Make sure you speak clearly and at a normal rate. Incorporate visual aids that have images or descriptive words. Repeat comments or questions made by the student's classmates. This helps all students alike. Check for understanding by asking students to repeat directions or demonstrate a skill. If an interpreter is involved, make sure to speak directly to the student, rather than the interpreter.

Visual Impairments

Children with visual impairments can play all of the same sports as their sighted peers, with some modifications. This may include a beeping ball or allowing blind player to walk around and feel the environment before they begin. Modifications can be made continuously until the best solution is found. Children with visual impairments and blindness may need more instruction and practice time to learn new concepts and movements. It is suggested that students receive pre-teaching before the start of a new unit. This can be done before school, after school, during orientation, or at home. Peer tutors may also be effective for students with visual impairments or blindness.

Adaptive Physical Education

Adaptive Physical Education (APE) is a direct service that can be provided to a special needs child, should the Committee on Preschool Special Education (CPSE) or the Committee on Special Education (CSE) determine that the child is in need of such service. In many cases, if a child is identified as visually impaired, physically handicapped, severely multiply impaired, or other health impaired, he or she will be warranted APE services.

Adaptive Physical Education (APE) is an adapted, or modified, physical education program designed to meet the individualized gross motor needs, or other disability-related challenges, of an identified student. The program can be provided one-on-one, in a small group, or within the general physical education setting. The APE instructor needs to be trained in assessing and working with special needs children. Lesson plans, rubrics, and worksheets need to be adapted for the needs of the children.

The need for Adaptive Physical Education (APE) is determined by the CPSE or CSE. The APE instructor assesses the child and presents the information to the committee. The assessment must include diagnostic and curriculum-based data, observations, and input by the child's general physical education teacher. If the child is receiving OT, PT or Vision Therapy (VT), then input should be obtained by these providers as well.

Based on the assessment and any other information provided by committee members, the committee determines whether or not APE services are needed. If the committee recommends such services, then APE becomes a part of the child's Individualized Education Plan (IEP). The plan must include the assessment information, the amount of APE to be received, whether or not the child will be in the general physical education setting, and goals with measurable objectives/ benchmarks.

It's important to note that APE should not be viewed as a related service. Because physical education is federally mandated for all students, the APE teacher is a direct service provider. The APE teacher is to provide adaptations or modifications that will allow the special needs child to participate in age-appropriate physical educational activities. Adaptations or modifications can be made in four areas:

1. Instruction. Rules, lesson plans, strategies, etc. can be modified or included to help the child be successful in physical education. For example, a down's syndrome child may respond to one word signs as reminders for doing a summersault correctly.

2. Rules. A rule can be adapted or changed if it allows the special needs child to be successful. For example, if the students are working on volley ball skills, a wheelchair bound student is allowed to serve the volley ball from four feet ahead of the serving line.

3. Equipment. Standard gym equipment can be replaced with other objects that vary in shape, color, size, etc. For example, when playing kickball, provide a large bright orange ball for a visually impaired child to kick.

4. Environment. If need be, change the size of the playing area or use tape to define the area. For example, if the general education students are pitching softballs back and forth, work with a severely mentally handicapped child on rolling a ball back and forth by starting out being two feet apart and gradually increasing the space.

For some special needs students, Adaptive Physical Education may be needed every school year. For other students, as they continue to make gains with their gross motor skills, APE services might be tapered back and at some point no longer needed. APE students need to be encouraged to do their best. Programs, such as the Special Olympics, have provided a wonderful and positive opportunity for APE students to experience competing just like their non-disabled peers.

Physical Exercise

Physical exercise is the performance of some activity in order to develop or maintain physical fitness and overall health.

It is often directed toward also honing athletic ability or skill.

Frequent and regular physical exercise is an important component in the prevention of some diseases such as heart disease, cardiovascular disease, Type 2 diabetes and obesity.

Physical exercise is considered important for maintaining physical fitness including healthy weight; building and maintaining healthy bones, muscles, and joints; promoting physiological well-being; reducing surgical risks; and strengthening the immune system.

Exercise and physical activity fall into four basic categories—endurance, strength, balance, and flexibility. Most people tend to focus on one activity or type of exercise and think they're doing enough. Each type is different, though. Doing them all will give you more benefits. Mixing it up also helps to reduce boredom and cut your risk of injury.

Though we've described each type separately, some activities fit into more than one category. For example, many endurance activities also build strength. Strength exercises also help improve balance.

Endurance

Endurance, or aerobic, activities increase your breathing and heart rate. They keep your heart, lungs, and circulatory system healthy and improve your overall fitness. Building your endurance makes it easier to carry out many of your everyday activities.

- Brisk walking or jogging
- Yard work (mowing, raking, digging)
- Dancing

Strength

Strength exercises make your muscles stronger. They may help you stay independent and carry out everyday activities, such as climbing stairs and carrying groceries. These exercises also are called "strength training" or "resistance training."

- Lifting weights
- Using a resistance band
- Using your own body weight

Balance

Balance exercises help prevent falls, a common problem in older adults. Many lower-body strength exercises also will improve your balance.

- Standing on one foot
- Heel-to-toe walk
- Tai Chi

Flexibility

Flexibility exercises stretch your muscles and can help your body stay limber. Being flexible gives you more freedom of movement for other exercises as well as for your everyday activities.

- Shoulder and upper arm stretch
- Calf stretch
- Yoga

Health Effects

Physical exercise is important for maintaining physical fitness and can contribute to maintaining a healthy weight, regulating digestive health, building and maintaining healthy bone density, muscle strength, and joint mobility, promoting physiological well-being, reducing surgical risks, and strengthening the immune system. Some studies indicate that exercise may increase life expectancy and the overall quality of life. People who participate in moderate to high levels of physical exercise have a lower mortality rate compared to individuals who by comparison are not physically active. Moderate levels of exercise have been correlated with preventing aging by reducing inflammatory potential. The majority of the benefits from exercise are achieved with around 3500 metabolic equivalent (MET) minutes per week. For example, climbing stairs 10 minutes, vacuuming 15 minutes, gardening 20 minutes, running 20 minutes, and walking or bicycling for transportation

25 minutes on a daily basis would *together* achieve about 3000 MET minutes a week. A lack of physical activity causes approximately 6% of the burden of disease from coronary heart disease, 7% of type 2 diabetes, 10% of breast cancer and 10% of colon cancer worldwide. Overall, physical inactivity causes 9% of premature mortality worldwide.

Fitness

Individuals can increase fitness following increases in physical activity levels. Increases in muscle size from resistance training is primarily determined by diet and testosterone. This genetic variation in improvement from training is one of the key physiological differences between elite athletes and the larger population. Studies have shown that exercising in middle age leads to better physical ability later in life.

Early motor skills and development have also shown to be related to physical activity and performance later in life. Children who have more proficient motor skills early on are more inclined to being physically active, and thus tend to perform well in sports and have better fitness levels. Early motor proficiency has a positive correlation to childhood physical activity and fitness levels, while less proficiency in motor skills results in a tendency to partake in a more sedentary lifestyle.

A 2015 meta-analysis demonstrated that high intensity training improved stamina more than lower intensity endurance training.

Cardiovascular System

The beneficial effect of exercise on the cardiovascular system is well documented. There is a direct correlation between physical inactivity and cardiovascular mortality, and physical inactivity is an independent risk factor for the development of coronary artery disease. Low levels of physical exercise increase the risk of cardiovascular diseases mortality.

Children who participate in physical exercise experience greater loss of body fat and increased cardiovascular fitness. Studies have shown that academic stress in youth increases the risk of cardiovascular disease in later years; however, these risks can be greatly decreased with regular physical exercise. There is a dose-response relation between the amount of exercise performed from approximately 700–2000 kcal of energy expenditure per week and all-cause mortality and cardiovascular disease mortality in middle-aged and elderly populations. The greatest potential for reduced mortality is in the sedentary who become moderately active. Studies have shown that since heart disease is the leading cause of death in women, regular exercise in aging women leads to healthier cardiovascular profiles. Most beneficial effects of physical activity on cardiovascular disease mortality can be attained through moderate-intensity activity (40–60% of maximal oxygen uptake, depending on age). Persons who modify their behavior after myocardial infarction to include regular exercise have improved rates of survival. Persons who remain sedentary have the highest risk for all-cause and cardiovascular disease mortality. According to the American Heart Association, exercise reduces the risk of cardiovascular diseases, including heart attack and stroke.

Immune System

Although there have been hundreds of studies on physical exercise and the immune system, there is little direct evidence on its connection to illness. Epidemiological evidence suggests that moderate exercise has a beneficial effect on the human immune system; an effect which is modeled in a J curve. Moderate exercise has been associated with a 29% decreased incidence of upper respiratory tract infections (URTI), but studies of marathon runners found that their prolonged high-intensity exercise was associated with an increased risk of infection occurrence. However, another study did not find the effect. Immune cell functions are impaired following acute sessions of prolonged, high-intensity exercise, and some studies have found that athletes are at a higher risk for infections. Studies have shown that strenuous stress for long durations, such as training for a marathon, can suppress the immune system by decreasing the concentration of lymphocytes. The immune systems of athletes and nonathletes are generally similar. Athletes may have slightly elevated natural killer cell count and cytolytic action, but these are unlikely to be clinically significant.

Vitamin C supplementation has been associated with lower incidence of upper respiratory tract infections in marathon runners.

Biomarkers of inflammation such as C-reactive protein, which are associated with chronic diseases, are reduced in active individuals relative to sedentary individuals, and the positive effects of exercise may be due to its anti-inflammatory effects. In individuals with heart disease, exercise interventions lower blood levels of fibrinogen and C-reactive protein, an important cardiovascular risk marker. The depression in the immune system following acute bouts of exercise may be one of the mechanisms for this anti-inflammatory effect.

Cancer

A systematic review evaluated 45 studies that examined the relationship between physical activity and cancer survivorship. According to the study results "There was consistent evidence from 27 observational studies that physical activity is associated with reduced all-cause, breast cancer–specific, and colon cancer–specific mortality".

Epigenetic Effects

Physical exercise was correlated with a lower methylation frequency of two tumor suppressor genes, CACNA2D3 and L3MBTL. Hypermethylation of CACNA2D3 is associated with gastric cancer, while hypermethylation of L3MBTL is associated with breast cancer, brain tumors and hematological malignancies. A recent study indicates that exercise results in reduced DNA methylation at CpG sites on genes associated with breast cancer.

Cancer Cachexia

Physical exercise is becoming a widely accepted non-pharmacological intervention for the prevention and attenuation of cancer cachexia. "Cachexia is a multiorganic syndrome associated with cancer, characterized by inflammation, body weight loss (at least 5%) and muscle and adipose tissue wasting". Exercise triggers the activation of the transcriptional coactivator peroxisome proliferator-activated receptor gamma coactivator-1α (PGC-1α), which suppresses FoxO- and NF-κB-dependent gene transcription during muscle atrophy that is induced by fasting or denervation; thus, PGC-1α may be a key intermediate responsible for the beneficial antiatrophic effects of physical exercise on cancer cachexia. The exercise-induced isoform PGC-1α4, which can repress myostatin and induce IGF1 and hypertrophy, is a potential drug target for treatment of cancer cachexia. Other factors, such as JUNB and SIRT1, that maintain skeletal muscle mass and promote hypertrophy are also induced with regular physical exercise.

Neurobiological

The neurobiological effects of physical exercise are numerous and involve a wide range of interrelated effects on brain structure, brain function, and cognition. A large body of research in humans has demonstrated that consistent aerobic exercise (e.g., 30 minutes every day) induces persistent improvements in certain cognitive functions, healthy alterations in gene expression in the brain, and beneficial forms of neuroplasticity and behavioral plasticity; some of these long-term effects include: increased neuron growth, increased neurological activity (e.g., c-Fos and BDNF signaling), improved stress coping, enhanced cognitive control of behavior, improved declarative, spatial, and working memory, and structural and functional improvements in brain structures and pathways associated with cognitive control and memory. The effects of exercise on cognition have important implications for improving academic performance in children and college students, improving adult productivity, preserving cognitive function in old age, preventing or treating certain neurological disorders, and improving overall quality of life.

In healthy adults, aerobic exercise has been shown to induce transient effects on cognition after a single exercise session and persistent effects on cognition following regular exercise over the course of several months. People who regularly perform aerobic exercise (e.g., running, jogging, brisk walking, swimming, and cycling) have greater scores on neuropsychological function and performance tests that measure certain cognitive functions, such as attentional control, inhibitory control, cognitive flexibility, working memory updating and capacity, declarative memory, spatial memory, and information processing speed. The transient effects of exercise on cognition include improvements in most executive functions (e.g., attention, working memory, cognitive flexibility, inhibitory control, problem solving, and decision making) and information processing speed for a period of up to 2 hours after exercising.

Aerobic exercise induces short- and long-term effects on mood and emotional states by promoting positive affect, inhibiting negative affect, and decreasing the biological response to acute psychological stress. Over the short-term, aerobic exercise functions as both an antidepressant and euphoriant, whereas consistent exercise produces general improvements in mood and self-esteem.

Regular aerobic exercise improves symptoms associated with a variety of central nervous system disorders and may be used as an adjunct therapy for these disorders. There is clear evidence of exercise treatment efficacy for major depressive disorder and attention deficit hyperactivity disorder. The American Academy of Neurology's clinical practice guideline for mild cognitive impairment indicates that clinicians should recommend regular exercise (two times per week) to individuals who have been diagnosed with this condition. Reviews of clinical evidence also support the use of exercise as an adjunct therapy for certain neurodegenerative disorders, particularly Alzheimer's disease and Parkinson's disease. Regular exercise is also associated with a lower risk of developing neurodegenerative disorders. A large body of preclinical evidence and emerging clinical evidence supports the use of exercise therapy for treating and preventing the development of drug addictions. Regular exercise has also been proposed as an adjunct therapy for brain cancers.

Depression

A number of medical reviews have indicated that exercise has a marked and persistent antidepressant effect in humans, an effect believed to be mediated through enhanced BDNF signaling in the brain. Several systematic reviews have analyzed the potential for physical exercise in the treatment of depressive disorders. The 2013 Cochrane Collaboration review on physical exercise for depression noted that, based upon limited evidence, it is more effective than a control intervention and comparable to psychological or antidepressant drug therapies. Three subsequent 2014 systematic reviews that included the Cochrane review in their analysis concluded with similar findings: one indicated that physical exercise is effective as an adjunct treatment (i.e., treatments that are used together) with antidepressant medication; the other two indicated that physical exercise has marked antidepressant effects and recommended the inclusion of physical activity as an adjunct treatment for mild–moderate depression and mental illness in general. One systematic review noted that yoga may be effective in alleviating symptoms of prenatal depression. Another review asserted that evidence from clinical trials supports the efficacy of physical exercise as a treatment for depression over a 2–4 month period.

A 2015 review of clinical evidence which included a medical guideline for the treatment of depression with exercise noted that the available evidence on the effectiveness of exercise therapy for depression suffers from some limitations; nonetheless, it stated that there is clear evidence of efficacy for reducing symptoms of depression. The review also noted that patient characteristics, the type of depressive disorder, and the nature of the exercise program all affect the antidepressant properties of exercise therapy. A meta-analysis from July 2016 concluded that physical exercise improves overall quality of life in individuals with depression relative to controls.

Continuous aerobic exercise can induce a transient state of euphoria, colloquially known as a "runner's high" in distance running or a "rower's high" in crew, through the increased biosynthesis of at least three euphoriant neurochemicals: anandamide (an endocannabinoid), β-endorphin (an endogenous opioid), and phenethylamine (a trace amine and amphetamine analog).

Sleep

A 2010 review of published scientific research suggested that exercise generally improves sleep for most people, and helps sleep disorders such as insomnia. The optimum time to exercise *may* be 4 to 8 hours before bedtime, though exercise at any time of day is beneficial, with the possible exception of heavy exercise taken shortly before bedtime, which may disturb sleep. There is, in any case, insufficient evidence to draw detailed conclusions about the relationship between exercise and sleep.

According to a 2005 study, exercise is the most recommended alternative to sleeping pills for resolving insomnia. Sleeping pills are more costly than to make time for a daily routine of staying fit, and may have dangerous side effects in the long run. Exercise can be a healthy, safe and inexpensive way to achieve more and better sleep.

Excessive Exercise

Too much exercise can be harmful. Without proper rest, the chance of stroke or other circulation problems increases, and muscle tissue may develop slowly. Extremely intense, long-term cardiovascular exercise, as can be seen in athletes who train for multiple marathons, has been associated with scarring of the heart and heart rhythm abnormalities. Specifically, high cardiac output has been shown to cause enlargement of the left and right ventricle volumes, increased ventricle wall thickness, and greater cardiac mass. These changes further result in myocardial cell damage in the lining of the heart, leading to scar tissue and thickened walls. During these processes, the protein troponin increases in the bloodstream, indicating cardiac muscle cell death and increased stress on the heart itself.

Inappropriate exercise can do more harm than good, with the definition of "inappropriate" varying according to the individual. For many activities, especially running and cycling, there are significant injuries that occur with poorly regimented exercise schedules. Injuries from accidents also remain a major concern, whereas the effects of increased exposure to air pollution seem only a minor concern.

In extreme instances, over-exercising induces serious performance loss. Unaccustomed overexertion of muscles leads to rhabdomyolysis (damage to muscle) most often seen in new army recruits. Another danger is overtraining, in which the intensity or volume of training exceeds the body's capacity to recover between bouts. One sign of Overtraining Syndrome (OTS) is suppressed immune function, with an increased incidence of upper respiratory tract infection (URTI). An increased incidence of URTIs is also associated with high volume/intensity training, as well as with excessive exercise (EE), such as in a marathon. Marathon training requires the runner to build their intensity week to week which makes them more susceptible to injury the more they increase their mileage. A study shows that in the last 10–15 years up to 90% of marathon runners have suffered a physical injury from their training.

Stopping excessive exercise suddenly may create a change in mood. Exercise should be controlled by each body's inherent limitations. While one set of joints and muscles may have the tolerance to withstand multiple marathons, another body may be damaged by 20 minutes of light jogging. This must be determined for each individual.

Too much exercise may cause a woman to miss her periods, a symptom known as amenorrhea. This is a very serious condition which indicates a woman is pushing her body beyond its natural boundaries.

Not only can excessive exercise cause physical damage, it can also cause psychological damage. Every athlete strives for perfection in their sport. This is what may begin their excessive exercising regime. If an athlete fails in this quest for perfection, this could result in anxiety, depression and low-self esteem. A study of 179 athletes, all of whom were Olympians or potential Olympians, was carried out in 2002 to find a relationship between perfectionism and sport-related competitive anxiety. It was found that athletes with lower self—esteem had higher personal standards and in comparison, those with high self-esteem had little concern in making mistakes or doubting themselves.

Mechanism of Effects

Skeletal Muscle

Resistance training and subsequent consumption of a protein-rich meal promotes muscle hypertrophy and gains in muscle strength by stimulating myofibrillar muscle protein synthesis

(MPS) and inhibiting muscle protein breakdown (MPB). The stimulation of muscle protein synthesis by resistance training occurs via phosphorylation of the mechanistic target of rapamycin (mTOR) and subsequent activation of mTORC1, which leads to protein biosynthesis in cellular ribosomes via phosphorylation of mTORC1's immediate targets (the p70S6 kinase and the translation repressor protein 4EBP1). The suppression of muscle protein breakdown following food consumption occurs primarily via increases in plasma insulin. Similarly, increased muscle protein synthesis (via activation of mTORC1) and suppressed muscle protein breakdown (via insulin-independent mechanisms) has also been shown to occur following ingestion of β-hydroxy β-methylbutyric acid.

Aerobic exercise induces mitochondrial biogenesis and an increased capacity for oxidative phosphorylation in the mitochondria of skeletal muscle, which is one mechanism by which aerobic exercise enhances submaximal endurance performance. These effects occur via an exercise-induced increase in the intracellular AMP:ATP ratio, thereby triggering the activation of AMP-activated protein kinase (AMPK) which subsequently phosphorylates peroxisome proliferator-activated receptor gamma coactivator-1α (PGC-1α), the master regulator of mitochondrial biogenesis.

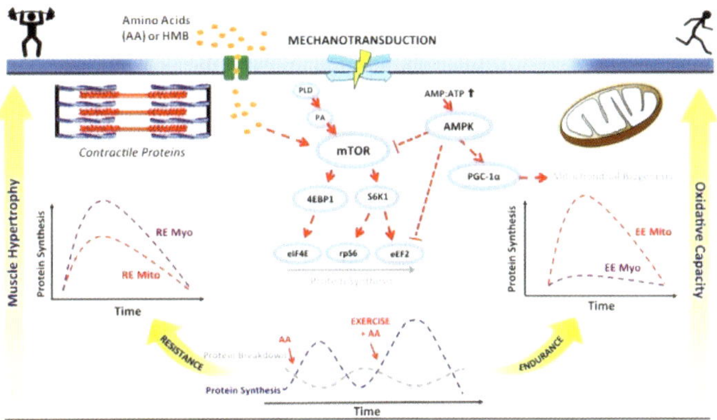

Diagram of the molecular signaling cascades that are involved in myofibrillar muscle protein synthesis and mitochondrial biogenesis in response to physical exercise and specific amino acids or their derivatives (primarily L-leucine and HMB).

Abbreviations and Representations

- PLD: phospholipase D
- PA: phosphatidic acid
- mTOR: mechanistic target of rapamycin
- AMP: adenosine monophosphate
- ATP: adenosine triphosphate
- AMPK: AMP-activated protein kinase
- PGC-1α: peroxisome proliferator-activated receptor gamma coactivator-1α
- S6K1: p70S6 kinase

- 4EBP1: eukaryotic translation initiation factor 4E-binding protein 1
- eIF4E: eukaryotic translation initiation factor 4E
- RPS6: ribosomal protein S6
- eEF2: eukaryotic elongation factor 2
- RE: resistance exercise; EE: endurance exercise
- Myo: myofibrillar; Mito: mitochondrial
- AA: amino acids
- HMB: β-hydroxy β-methylbutyric acid
- ↑ represents activation
- T represents inhibition

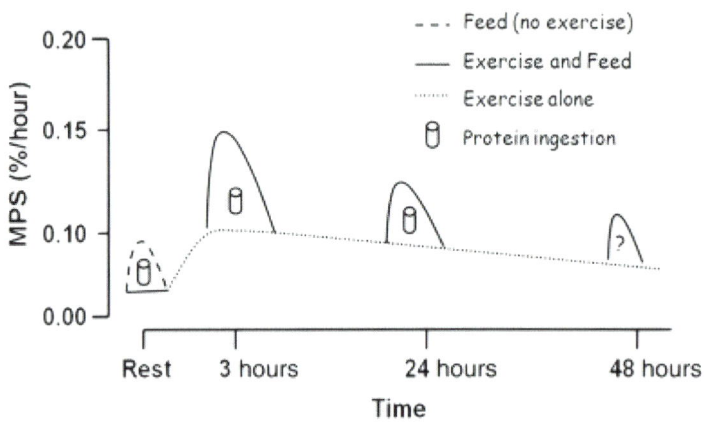

Resistance training stimulates muscle protein synthesis (MPS) for a period of up to 48 hours following exercise (shown by dotted line). Ingestion of a protein-rich meal at any point during this period will augment the exercise-induced increase in muscle protein synthesis (shown by solid lines).

Other Peripheral Organs

Developing research has demonstrated that many of the benefits of exercise are mediated through the role of skeletal muscle as an endocrine organ. That is, contracting muscles release multiple substances known as myokines which promote the growth of new tissue, tissue repair, and multiple anti-inflammatory functions, which in turn reduce the risk of developing various inflammatory diseases. Exercise reduces levels of cortisol, which causes many health problems, both physical and mental. Endurance exercise before meals lowers blood glucose more than the same exercise after meals. There is evidence that vigorous exercise (90–95% of VO_2 max) induces a greater degree of physiological cardiac hypertrophy than moderate exercise (40 to 70% of VO_2 max), but it is unknown whether this has any effects on overall morbidity and/or mortality. Both aerobic and anaerobic exercise work to increase the mechanical efficiency of the heart by increasing cardiac volume (aerobic exercise), or myocardial thickness (strength training). Ventricular hypertrophy, the thickening of the ventricular walls, is generally beneficial and healthy if it occurs in response to exercise.

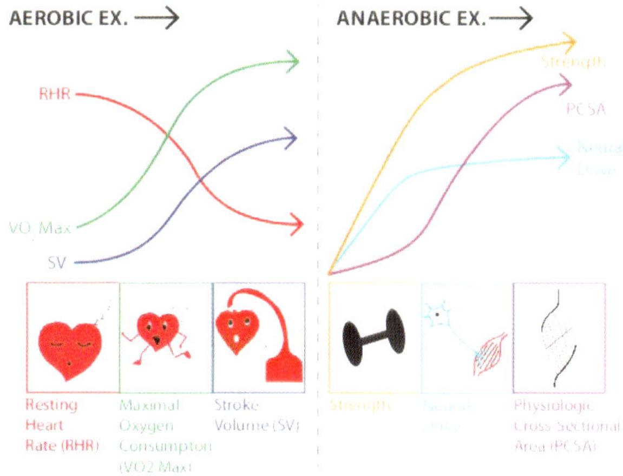

Summary of long-term adaptations to regular aerobic and anaerobic exercise.

Aerobic exercise can cause several central cardiovascular adaptations, including an increase in stroke volume (SV) and maximal aerobic capacity (VO_2 max), as well as a decrease in resting heart rate (RHR). Long-term adaptations to resistance training, the most common form of anaerobic exercise, include muscular hypertrophy, an increase in the physiological cross-sectional area (PCSA) of muscle(s), and an increase in neural drive, both of which lead to increased muscular strength. Neural adaptations begin more quickly and plateau prior to the hypertrophic response.

Central Nervous System

The effects of physical exercise on the central nervous system are mediated in part by specific neurotrophic factor hormones that are released into the blood stream by muscles, including BDNF, IGF-1, and VEGF.

Public Health Measures

Multiple component community-wide campaigns are frequently used in an attempt to increase a population's level of physical activity. A 2015 Cochrane review, however, did not find evidence supporting a benefit. The quality of the underlying evidence was also poor. However, there is some evidence that school-based interventions can increase activity levels and fitness in children. Another Cochrane review found some evidence that certain types of exercise programmes, such as those involving gait, balance, co-ordination and functional tasks, can improve balance in older adults. Following progressive resistance training, older adults also respond with improved physical function. Survey of brief interventions promoting physical activity found that they are cost-effective, although there are variations between studies.

Environmental approaches appear promising: signs that encourage the use of stairs, as well as community campaigns, may increase exercise levels. The city of Bogotá, Colombia, for example, blocks off 113 kilometers (70 mi) of roads on Sundays and holidays to make it easier for its citizens to get exercise. Such pedestrian zones are part of an effort to combat chronic diseases and to maintain a healthy BMI.

To identify which public health strategies are effective, a Cochrane overview of reviews is in preparation.

Physical exercise was said to decrease healthcare costs, increase the rate of job attendance, as well as increase the amount of effort women put into their jobs. There is some level of concern about additional exposure to air pollution when exercising outdoors, especially near traffic.

Children will mimic the behavior of their parents in relation to physical exercise. Parents can thus promote physical activity and limit the amount of time children spend in front of screens.

Overweight children who participate in physical exercise experience greater loss of body fat and increased cardiovascular fitness. According to the Centers for Disease Control and Prevention in the United States, both children and adults should do 60 minutes or more of physical activity each day. Implementing physical exercise in the school system and ensuring an environment in which children can reduce barriers to maintain a healthy lifestyle is essential.

The European Commission - DG EAC - Directorate General for Education and Culture - has dedicated programs and funds for HEPA - Health Enhancing Physical Activity projects within its Horizon 2020 and Erasmus+ program, as research showed that too many Europeans are not physically active enough. Financing is available for increased collaboration between players active in this field across the EU and around the world, the promotion of HEPA in the EU and its partner countries and the European Sports Week. The DG EAC regularly publishes a Eurobarometer on sport and physical activity.

Exercise Trends

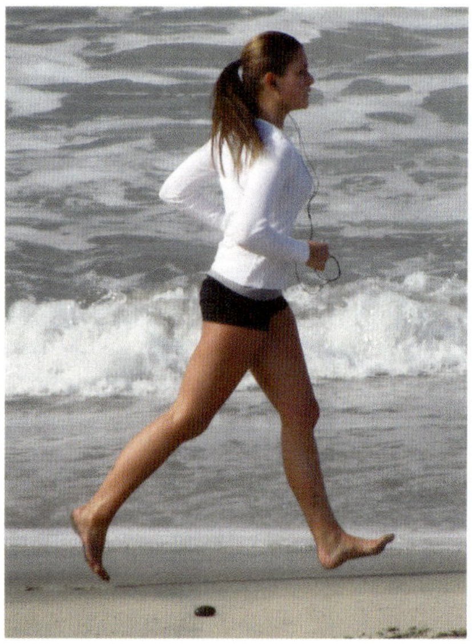

Running has become a popular form of exercise.

Worldwide there has been a large shift towards less physically demanding work. This has been accompanied by increasing use of mechanized transportation, a greater prevalence of labor saving technology in the home, and fewer active recreational pursuits. Personal lifestyle changes however can correct the lack of physical exercise.

Research in 2015 indicates integrating mindfulness to physical exercise interventions increases exercise adherence, self-efficacy and also has positive effects both psychologically and physiologically.

Social and Cultural Variation

Exercising looks different in every country, as do the motivations behind exercising. In some countries, people exercise primarily indoors, and in others, people exercise primarily outdoors. People may exercise for personal enjoyment, health and well-being, social interactions, competition or training, etc. These differences could potentially be attributed to geographic location, social tendencies, or otherwise.

In Colombia, citizens value and celebrate the outdoor environments of their country. In many instances, they utilize outdoor activities as social gatherings to enjoy nature and their communities. In Bogotá, Colombia, a 70-mile stretch of road known as the Ciclovía is shut down each Sunday for bicyclists, runners, rollerbladers, skateboarders and other exercisers to work out and enjoy their surroundings.

Similarly to Colombia, citizens of Cambodia tend to exercise socially outside. In this country, public gyms have become quite popular. People will congregate at these outdoor gyms not only to utilize the public facilities, but also to organize aerobics and dance sessions, which are open to the public.

Sweden has also begun developing outdoor gyms, called *utegym*. These gyms are free to the public and are often placed in beautiful, picturesque environments. People will swim in rivers, use boats, and run through forests to stay healthy and enjoy the natural world around them. This is especially possible in Sweden due to its geographical location.

Chinese exercise, particularly in the retired community, seems to be socially grounded. In the mornings, dances are held in public parks; these gatherings may include Latin dancing, ballroom dancing, tango, or even the jitterbug. Dancing in public allows people to interact with those with whom they would not normally interact, allowing for both health benefits and social benefits.

These sociocultural variations in physical exercise show how people in different geographic locations and social climates have varying motivations and methods of exercising. Physical exercise can improve health and well-being, as well as enhance community ties and appreciation of natural beauty.

Nutrition and Recovery

Proper nutrition is as important to health as exercise. When exercising, it becomes even more important to have a good diet to ensure that the body has the correct ratio of macronutrients while providing ample micronutrients, in order to aid the body with the recovery process following strenuous exercise.

Active recovery is recommended after participating in physical exercise because it removes lactate from the blood more quickly than inactive recovery. Removing lactate from circulation allows for an easy decline in body temperature, which can also benefit the immune system, as an individual may be vulnerable to minor illnesses if the body temperature drops too abruptly after physical exercise.

Calisthenics

The word calisthenics comes from the Greek ancient words: kalos (which means beauty) and sthenos (which means strength).These ancient words give a good representation of what calisthenics is. There is an element of beauty, not only because of the beautiful body that you can shape through the practice - but also because of how aesthetically pleasing the more advanced calisthenics exercises are. Experienced practitioners often aim to reach perfect form, resulting in what looks like gravity-defying endeavors to those who are not familiar to the art.

Basically calisthenics is a fancy word for bodyweight training.

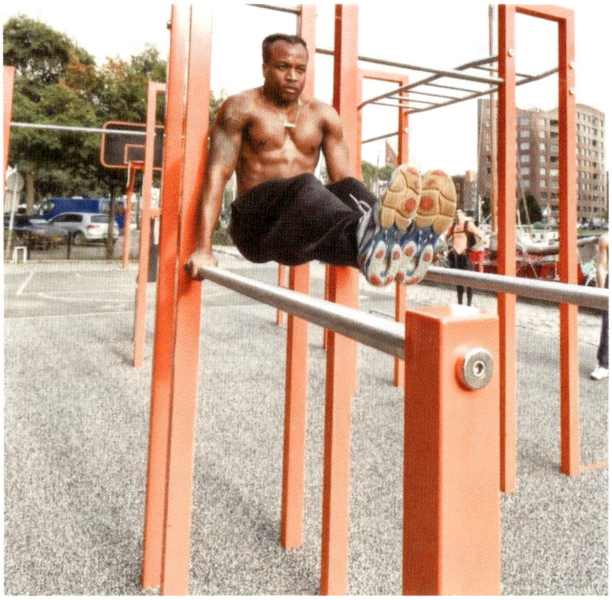

Calisthenic training involves any exercises performed using no added weight, and is commonly referred to as body-weight training. Calisthenic training can be done as a stand-alone routine, or programmed into any weight loss, bodybuilding or fitness workout. It has many benefits and is convenient, and it can be tailored to suit beginner, intermediate or advanced trainees.

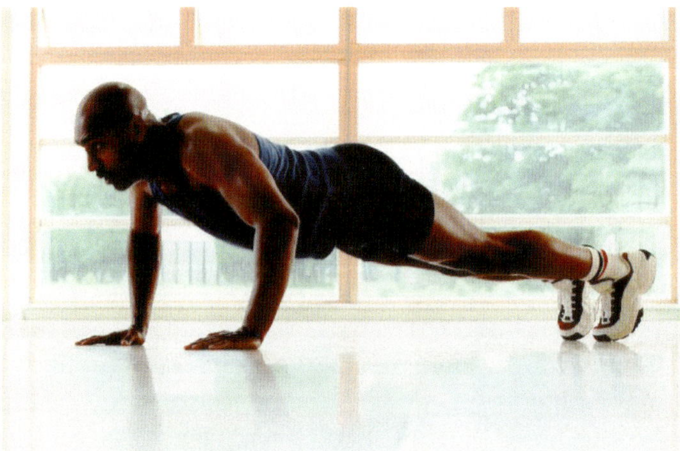

Upper-Body Exercises

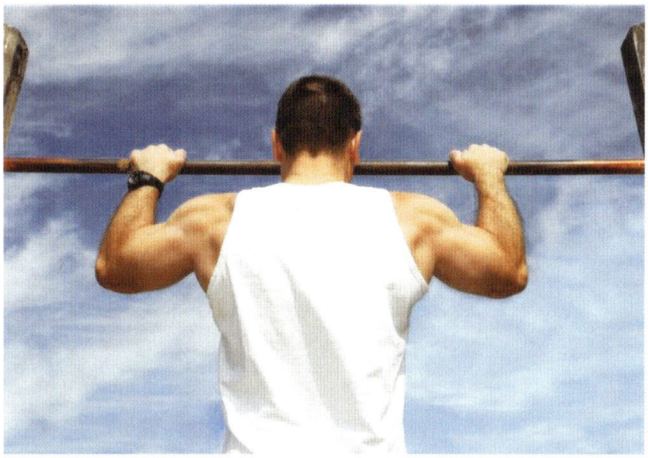

The most well-known upper-body calisthenic exercises are pushups and pullups. Pushups are great for building muscle in your chest, shoulders and triceps muscles, as well as improving your core stability and muscular endurance. Pullups work your back, biceps and grip, and are a great test of upper-body strength. For pullups, try changing your grip width, or use a tree branch or pair of gymnastic rings for an extra challenge.

Lower-Body Exercises

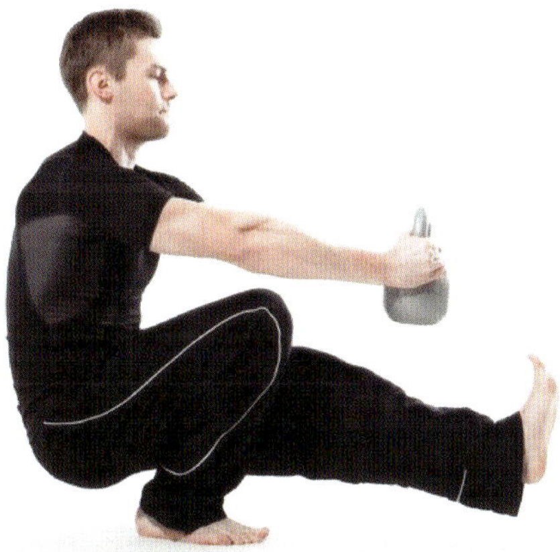

One of the most effective lower-body calisthenics is the squat. Stand with your feet slightly wider than shoulder-width apart, and your toes turned out about 10 degrees. Squat down by pushing your hips back and knees out, until you can go no lower, then stand back up again. You can perform different variations of the squat to get a whole lower-body workout. Change your foot placement and speed, or try Tabata squats, where you perform as many repetitions as you can in 20 seconds, rest for 10 seconds, then repeat for another seven rounds. One-legged squats, known as pistols, are a challenging variation that can increase your lower-body strength, balance and mobility. Lunges, in which you take a large step forward, and then lower your body until your front leg is parallel to the floor, are another effective body-weight calisthenic. This exercise targets your quads but uses a number of other muscles.

Common Exercises

In addition to the various stretches, some of the more common calisthenic exercises include:

- Muscle-ups

  One of the basic calisthenics routines. Performed by a combination routine of a pull-up followed by a dip. May be done on pullup bars or rings.

- Squat jumps ("Toyota jumps"/box jumps)

  Performed by entering a squatting position, then using a plyometric jumping movement to jump as high as possible.

- Front lever

  A front lever is performed by lowering from an inverted hang until the body is completely horizontal and straight with the front of the body facing upwards. May be done on rings or pull-up bar.

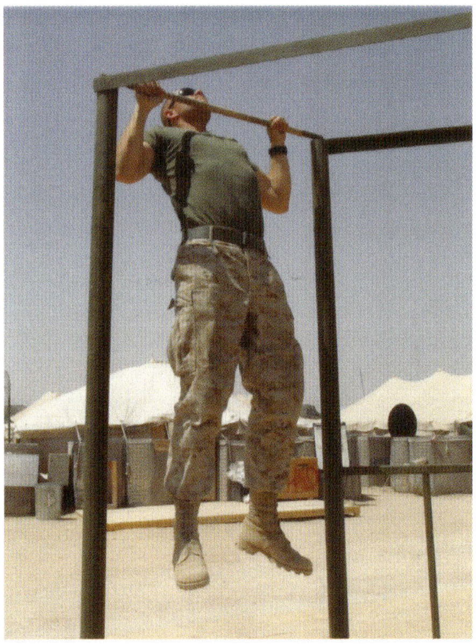

A US Marine performs a pull-up, a common calisthenic exercise.

- Push-ups

  Performed face down on the floor, palms against floor under the shoulders, toes curled upwards against the floor. The arms are used to lift the body while maintaining a straight line from head to heel. The arms of the subject should go from fully extended in the high position to nearly fully flexed in the low position, while the subject makes sure to avoid resting on the floor. Resting is only done in the high position of the exercise. Chest, shoulders, and triceps are trained with this exercise. By furthering the range of motion, what is often called a push up, by pushing the shoulders downwards at the top the serratus anterior comes further into play.

- Pull-ups

An overhead bar (sometimes called a chin-up bar) is grasped using a shoulder-width grip. The subject lifts their body up, chin level with the bar, and keeping the back straight throughout. The bar remains in front of the subject at all times. The subject then slowly returns to starting position in a slow controlled manner. This primarily trains the lats or upper back muscles, as well as the forearms. An underhand grip variation or chin-up trains both the back and biceps.

- Chin-ups

Much like the pull-up, except that the hand placement is reversed. The hands are facing the person as he pulls his body up using the chin-up bar. The chin-up focuses on the biceps muscles, rather than the Latissimus dorsi muscle which is the focus of the pull up.

- Squats

Standing with feet shoulder width apart, the subject squats down as far as possible, bringing the arms forward parallel to the floor. The subject then returns to standing position. Squats train the quadriceps, hamstrings, calves, and gluteal muscles.

- Back lever

A back lever is performed by lowering from an inverted hang from rings or bar, until the gymnast's body is parallel to the ground and facing towards the floor.

- Handstand

A handstand is the act of supporting the body in a stable, inverted vertical position by balancing on the hands. In a basic handstand the body is held straight with arms and legs fully extended, with hands spaced approximately shoulder-width apart.

- Dips

Done between parallel bars or facing either direction of trapezoid bars found in some gyms. Feet are crossed with either foot in front and the body is lowered until the elbows are in line with the shoulders. The subject then pushes up until the arms are fully extended, but without locking the elbows. Dips focus primarily on the chest, triceps, and deltoids, especially the anterior portion.

- Hyperextensions

Performed in a prone position on the ground, the individual raises the legs, arms and upper body off the ground.

- Leg raises

Lying on the back, hands in fists under buttocks, move feet up and down.

- Planks

This is the name for holding the 'top' position of a push-up for extended periods of time. The primary muscle involved in this exercise is the rectus abdominis.

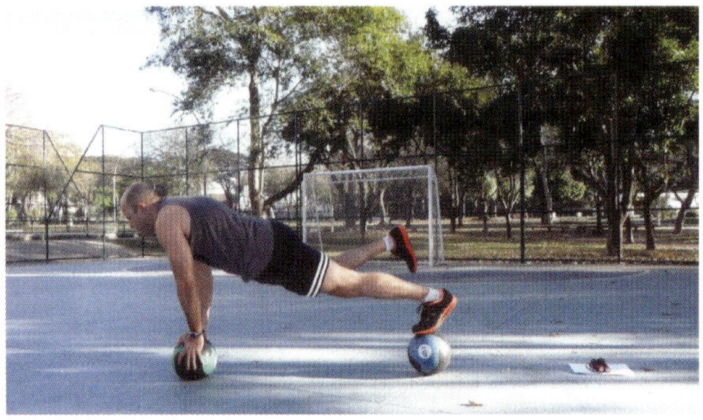

Plank on medicine balls

- Shuttle runs

  This is running back and forth between two points (or cones) typically separated by 5-40 meters, as fast as possible, with a touchdown. The emphasis should be on stopping, turning back and accelerate back to a sprint as quickly as possible.

- Burpees

  A full body calisthenics workout that works abdominal muscles, chest, arms, legs, and some parts of the back.

Calisthenics Parks

Especially for calisthenics training there is a rising amount of centralized outdoor fitness training areas. These calisthenics parks are central modules with equipment like pull up bars, monkey bar, parallel bar and wall bars at one location. The bars are connected to enable transfers between the elements.

Benefits of Calisthenics Workouts

You don't need any equipment. The beauty of calisthenics is that you can do it anywhere, anytime—all you need is your body. "It's one of the only ways to build mass and strength without the use of weights,".

You can build serious strength. You might be thinking: "How, if you're not hoisting barbells or dumbbells?" But you can accomplish a lot using just your own bodyweight, If you're a 150-lb woman doing a bodyweight pull-up, you're effectively lifting 150 lbs.

It's true that "you will reach a certain max point of muscle growth with calisthenics because muscle mass comes from progressive resistance, and there will only ever be so much resistance provided by your own body," but that's where getting creative comes into play. Use elevated surfaces to change the angle of exercises, increasing the percentage of bodyweight that you're lifting. Use vertical surfaces to challenge your body in new ways, and recruit your core like you wouldn't believe. Go faster, slower, longer, upside down, or increase your range of motion to keep provoking physical and mental adaptions.

You'll move better IRL. Since calisthenics is all about moving your body in space, it's the ultimate kind of functional movement training. "Functional training means training in a way that will directly enhance the way you perform everyday life tasks or particular physical requirements of your work or sport,"

You likely maintain better form. "When using free weights or machines, you can continue to progress your strength and muscle mass; however, people often end up using too much resistance on a machine or weights that are too heavy and that leads to compensating, meaning you don't execute the exercise properly using the correct muscles," Calisthenics gives you the necessary solid base of strength for when/if you do incorporate external resistance into your training. "If you can't lift your body weight you definitely shouldn't be trying to lift more on a machine."

You hit every. single. muscle. "Calisthenics involves using the entire body and not emphasizing certain muscles over others".

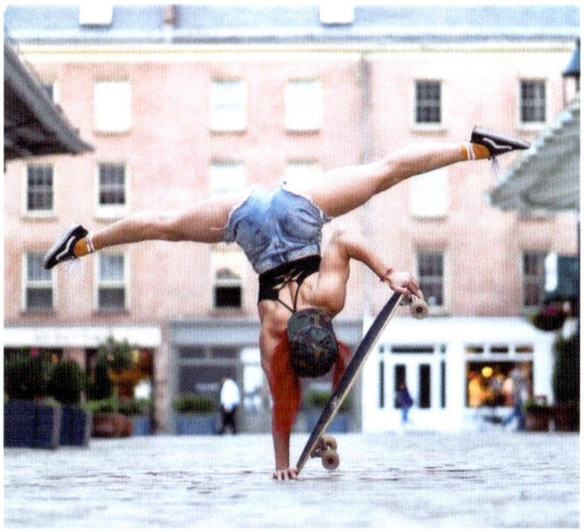

You'll be gentler on your joints and connective tissue. Resistance training—when performed incorrectly, with too-heavy weights, too often, or in a way that creates imbalances—can put extra stress on soft tissue structures like your tendons, ligaments, and fascia, Calisthenics, on the other hand, "only develops strength and size in proportion to your muscular system with authentic and natural movements."

You improve your brain-body connection. "Calisthenics training develops those fine motor skills that require your brain to work hard as well as your body," "Coordination, speed, power, acceleration, strength, quickness, and agility, are all actions that are demonstrated by a body trained in the art of calisthenics." Think of a gymnast: It takes a lot of strength, flexibility, and stamina to perform these movements, not to mention unbelievable coordination.

Anaerobic Exercise

While "aerobic" means "with oxygen," anaerobic means "without air" or "without oxygen." Anaerobic exercise is short-lasting, high-intensity activity, where your body's demand for oxygen exceeds the oxygen supply available. Anaerobic exercise relies on energy sources that are stored in the muscles and, unlike aerobic exercise, is not dependent on oxygen from (breathing) the air. Examples of anaerobic exercise include: heavy weight-lifting, all types of sprints (running, biking, etc.), jumping rope, hill climbing, interval training, isometrics, or any rapid burst of hard exercise.

Benefits

In addition to helping your body handle lactic acid effectively, anaerobic exercise has great benefits for your overall health. Anaerobic exercise:

- Builds and maintains lean muscle mass.
- Protects your joints. Increased muscle strength and muscle mass helps protect your joints, which can protect you from injury.
- Boosts metabolism. Anaerobic exercise helps boost metabolism because it helps build and maintain lean muscle. Lean muscle mass is metabolically active, so the more lean muscle mass you have, the more calories you will burn.
- Increases bone strength and density. Anaerobic activity will increase the strength and density of your bones more than any other type of exercise, therefore decreasing your risk of osteoporosis.
- Improves your energy. Your body relies on glycogen stored in your muscles as energy. Regular anaerobic exercise increases your body's ability to store glycogen, giving you more energy during intense physical activity.
- Increases sports performance. Regular anaerobic exercise increases strength, speed and power, which will ultimately help improve your sports performance.

Aerobic Exercise

Aerobic exercise which is primarily known as cardiovascular exercise or fat burning exercise is a rhythmic motion of more than one muscle groups in the body.

The reason why aerobic exercise is also known as fat burning exercise is that of its potential to use fat over carbohydrates as a fuel to keep you moving during a workout.

Aerobic exercise is any physical activity that makes you sweat, causes you to breathe harder, and gets your heart beating faster than at rest. It strengthens your heart and lungs and trains your cardiovascular system to manage and deliver oxygen more quickly and efficiently throughout your body. Aerobic exercise uses your large muscle groups, is rhythmic in nature, and can be maintained continuously for at least 10 minutes.

Types of Aerobic Exercise

1. Walking

Walking habit can improve your health. It gives you better cardiovascular fitness, stronger leg muscles, lower blood pressure, lower risk of heart disease, diabetes, bowel cancer and osteoporosis.

It's also a safe, low-impact exercise that most people can do — and it's especially good if you're overweight, unused to physical activity or pregnant.

Walking for 30 minutes a day at moderate intensity is great. Walking for a longer period of time is better still. As you get fitter, you will be able to walk more briskly. Walking up and down hills will also help to boost stamina and leg strength. You'll get even more benefits from a walk if you swing your arms as this helps you walk faster and can burn 5 to 10 percent more kilojoules.

- Running

  Like walking, running is an inexpensive exercise you can do anywhere at a time that suits you. It is beneficial in helping to improve heart and bone health. Its advantage over walking is that it improves heart fitness and burns kilojoules at a greater rate. It takes roughly an hour for a walker to burn the same number of kilojoules that a runner burns in 30 minutes.

  Jogging is running at a slower pace which is still a great aerobic exercise. Like walking, running or jogging can be a social activity you can do with a friend or in a group. Many areas have running clubs which welcome runners of all skill levels.

- Swimming

  If it's too hot to walk or run, swimming can be a cool way to get fit. It's a low-cost workout for the whole body especially the muscles of the back, shoulder and arms and improves flexibility as well. It's a good way to exercise if you're overweight, pregnant or have joint problems as the water helps support your weight and can reduce the pressure on your joints. The risk of injury to muscles, ligaments or joints is also low.

- Aquarobics

  These exercise sessions are done in a swimming pool and are available at some fitness centres or through local community health services. Aquarobics is a low-impact way to improve heart fitness and muscle strength without stressing the joints. It's particularly suitable for anyone who's pregnant, has joint problems and is overweight or unused to exercise.

- Cycling

  Cycling does double duty as an aerobic workout as well as being a low-cost, eco-friendly form of transport. It's good exercise for improving leg strength and toning leg and buttock muscles — but with less stress on joints compared to running or walking. If you'd rather not ride outdoors, exercise bikes at home or in a gym are a good alternative.

  Spinning classes available at some fitness centres are another indoor cycling option. These involve simulating different biking activities on a stationary bike — for example, cycling uphill or sprints — and are choreographed to music.

- Rowing

  Rowing is a low-impact alternative to running or cycling that can improve heart fitness and strengthen the muscles of the upper body, back and abdomen. You can enjoy rowing outdoors by joining a rowing club or hiring a rowboat, or indoors using a rowing machine at the gym or at home.

- Boxing

    This is a good aerobic workout that also boosts upper body strength — and helps you let off steam. Boxing classes are widely available in many gyms. Some classes involve sparring with a partner — you take it in turns to hold a pad or pads while the other person punches them while wearing boxing mitts. Others involve no mitts or pads, just air punching and other moves that simulate boxing training. You can also use a punching bag either at the gym or in your own home.

- Aerobic or 'cardio' classes

    Available in most gyms and community centres, these classes keep you moving to music using a variety of different exercises that raise your heart rate.

- Team sports

    Fast-paced sports such as soccer, netball or basketball provide an aerobic workout, improve muscle and bone strength — and provide a social activity as well.

- Dancing

    Faster styles of dancing such as jazz, hip hop, African and Latin American can provide an aerobic workout and improve flexibility and bone strength as well as being a lot of fun. It's also an indoor activity you can do in all weather conditions. Dancing classes are available in many community centres, gyms and dance schools.

Physical Fitness

Physical fitness is an important part of life. It is an indicator which shows whether you have the ability to perform and enjoy day to day physical activities with ease.

Physical fitness is generally achieved through -

- physical activity and exercise,
- correct nutrition,
- enough rest (good quality sleep),
- Stress management and relaxation.

Physical fitness is defined as the state of general well being, physically sound and healthy, along with mental stability.

Previously fitness was commonly defined as the capacity of the person to meet the physical demands of daily life and carry out the day's activities without undue fatigue.

However, because of increased leisure time, changes in lifestyles rendered this definition insufficient. These days, physical fitness is considered a measure of the body's ability to function efficiently and effectively in work and leisure activities, to be healthy, to resist hypo-kinetic diseases, and to meet emergency situations.

Health Related Fitness Components

These are

1. Body composition
2. Cardiovascular fitness
3. Flexibility
4. Muscular endurance
5. Muscle strength

Health Related Physical Fitness

What is Physical Fitness or what is Health Related Physical fitness? - It is best defined as activity aimed to improve your health. The goal of health related fitness is prevention of or rehabilitation from disease as well as the development of a high level of functional capacity for daily tasks.

Health related physical fitness is further divided into 5 parts i.e. components of health related physical fitness are:

1. Balanced Body Composition

In other words the ratio of fat to muscle. Minimum of fat and maximum of lean mass is a sign of a healthy and fit body.

2. Cardiovascular Fitness or Endurance

Cardiovascular endurance can be defined as the component which helps to determine if the heart and lungs are working in coordination. It shows the ability of the body to deliver oxygen and nutrients to tissues and to remove wastes.

Cardiovascular exercises or aerobics -walking, running, biking, rowing, treadmills

3. Flexibility

Flexibility can be defined as the component which checks the ability of the joints in the body to move to their full range of motion.

Flexibility exercises - stretching, yoga, Tai Chi

4. Muscular Endurance

Muscular endurance is defined as the ability of the body to perform repeated exercises without getting tired. If a person can perform more number of repetitions of a particular strength training exercise, then it can be said that he/she has good muscular endurance.

Strength training exercises such as running, jogging, cross-training on an elliptical machine, etc.

5. Muscle StrengTH

Muscle strength can be defined as the capability of the muscles to lift weight. By doing weight training exercises every alternate day increases the muscle mass of the body.

Weight training exercises - push ups, pull ups, biceps curls, pectoral fly, leg extensions, back extension, etc.

Skill related components of physical fitness:

1. Agility

2. Balance

3. Coordination

4. Power

5. Reaction Time

6. Speed

Physiological components of fitness:

1. Metabolic

2. Morphological

3. Bone integrity

4. Other

Sports related components of fitness:

1. Team sport

2. Individual sport

So what is physical fitness? It is a combination of all these fitness components mentioned above.

Physical fitness and wellness is far more attainable than commonly perceived. A good physical fitness and wellness can be described as a condition that helps individuals look, feel and do their best.

Physical fitness is not just about having a thin lean body frame, but it is about having cardiovascular and muscular endurance, strong immunity system, and most importantly, a satisfied, happy and well balanced state of mind.

Cardiorespiratory Fitness

Cardiorespiratory fitness is the ability of the body's circulatory and respiratory systems to supply fuel and oxygen during sustained physical activity. It is a good indicator of how much physical activity you routinely perform. It can be objectively measured in metabolic equivalents (METs) or maximal oxygen uptake (VO2 max) using treadmill or cycle ergometer tests or estimated by using simpler tests.

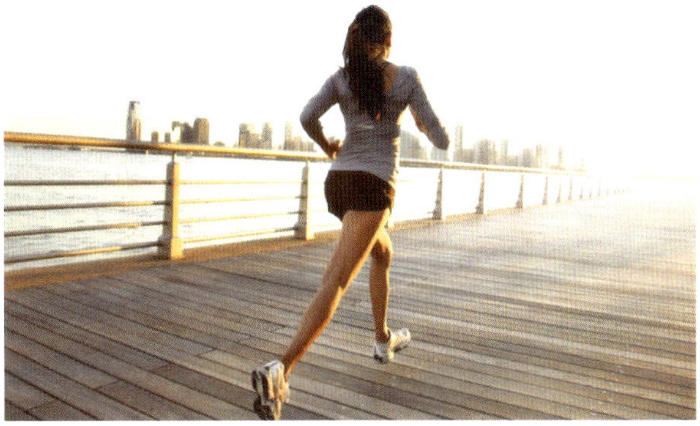

Cardiorespiratory fitness is an important health indicator and it can predict cardiovascular diseases mortality. Most people can improve it through regular physical activity.

Measurement of Cardiorespiratory Fitness

The best test of cardiorespiratory fitness is the peak oxygen uptake, VO2 max, and testing for it is used in research studies. But directly measuring this is difficult, it's usually done on a treadmill wearing breathing apparatus and hooked up to an ECG. That's not something you find in every gym. Instead, you will often perform a submaximal test that has been correlated with VO2 max.

Popular methods to measure your cardiorespiratory fitness include the 1-mile walk test. This is a simple test that requires only a stopwatch, a measured one-mile course (laps around a track is an easy choice), and a way to measure heart rate. It has been well-correlated to estimate VO2 max. It has advantages in that it can be performed by people who may not like to run.

The 12-minute run test is another popular submaximal test, developed by Dr. Ken Cooper and used by fitness trainers and the military. You warm up and then run or walk as far as you can in 12 minutes. You would need an accurate means to measure the distance, such as how many laps you were able to make around a track, but you don't need to take your heart rate.

With these tests, there are normal values by age and sex to compare yourself to. By taking a test before and after starting an exercise program, you can measure improvements.

Cardiovascular System

The cardiovascular system responds to changing demands on the body by adjusting cardiac output, blood flow, and blood pressure. Cardiac output is defined as the product of heart rate and stroke volume which represents the volume of blood being pumped by the heart each minute. Cardiac output increases during physical activity due to an increase in both the heart rate and stroke volume. At the beginning of exercise, the cardiovascular adaptations are very rapid: "Within a second after muscular contraction, there is a withdrawal of vagal outflow to the heart, which is followed by an increase in sympathetic stimulation of the heart. This results in an increase in cardiac output to ensure that blood flow to the muscle is matched to the metabolic needs". Both heart rate and stroke volume vary directly with the intensity of the exercise performed and many improvements can be made through continuous training.

Another important issue is the regulation of blood flow during exercise. Blood flow must increase in order to provide the working muscle with more oxygenated blood which can be accomplished through neural and chemical regulation. Blood vessels are under sympathetic tone; therefore, the release of noradrenaline and adrenaline will cause vasoconstriction of non-essential tissues such as the liver, intestines, and kidneys, and decrease neurotransmitter release to the active muscles promoting vasodilatation. Also, chemical factors such as a decrease in oxygen concentration and an increase in carbon dioxide or lactic acid concentration in the blood promote vasodilatation to increase blood flow. As a result of increased vascular resistance, blood pressure rises throughout exercise and stimulates baroreceptors in the carotid arteries and aortic arch. "These pressure receptors are important since they regulate arterial blood pressure around an elevated systemic pressure during exercise".

Respiratory System Adaptations

Although all of the described adaptations in the body to maintain homeostatic balance during exercise are very important, the most essential factor is the involvement of the respiratory system. The respiratory system allows for the proper exchange and transport of gases to and from the lungs while being able to control the ventilation rate through neural and chemical impulses. In addition, the body is able to efficiently use the three energy systems which include the phosphagen system, the glycolytic system, and the oxidative system.

Temperature Regulation

In most cases, as the body is exposed to physical activity, the core temperature of the body tends to rise as heat gain becomes larger than the amount of heat lost. "The factors that contribute to heat gain during exercise include anything that stimulate metabolic rate, anything from the external environment that causes heat gain, and the ability of the body to dissipate heat under any given set of circumstances". In response to an increase in core temperature, there are a variety of factors which adapt in order to help restore heat balance. The main physiological response to an increase in body temperature is mediated by the thermal regulatory center located in the hypothalamus of the brain which connects to thermal receptors and effectors. There are numerous thermal effectors including sweat glands, smooth muscles of blood vessels, some endocrine glands, and skeletal muscle. With an increase in the core temperature, the thermal regulatory center will stimulate the arterioles supplying blood to the skin to dilate along with the release of sweat on the skin surface to reduce temperature through evaporation. In addition to the involuntary regulation of temperature, the hypothalamus is able to communicate with the cerebral cortex to initiate voluntary control such as removing clothing or drinking cold water. With all regulations taken into account, the body is able to maintain core temperature within about two or three degrees Celsius during exercise.

It can be broken down into two components. The first component of cardiorespiratory fitness is the ability of your body to *transport oxygen* to your muscles during prolonged exercise. The second component of cardiorespiratory fitness is the ability of your muscles to *absorb and use oxygen* while you are exercising.

Your body's ability to *transport oxygen* to your muscles is dependent on the coordinated activities of your heart, arteries, veins, and lungs. The process works like this:

1. You breathe air into your lungs. The oxygen in the air you breathe is absorbed into the blood in the capillaries that surround your lungs and then transported via the pulmonary vein into the left side of your heart.
2. The oxygenated blood is pumped out of the left side of your heart and into the arteries that deliver it throughout your body to your muscles.
3. When the oxygenated blood reaches your muscles the oxygen is absorbed into your muscle cells from the blood capillaries that surround them. At the same time that your blood is providing oxygen to your muscles, it is also removing carbon dioxide, a waste product from muscle cellular respiration, from them. The now de-oxygenated and carbon dioxide rich blood is returned to the right side of your heart via your veins.
4. The de-oxygenated and carbon dioxide rich blood is pumped out of the right side of your heart to your lungs via your pulmonary artery. Once in the lungs, your blood releases the carbon dioxide into the air that you breathe out and absorbs more oxygen from the air that you breathe in, and the entire process begins again.

Therefore, your cardiorespiratory fitness level is in part (remember, there is a second component to cardiorespiratory fitness yet to be discussed) a measure of how well your heart, arteries, veins, and lungs are able to work together to transport oxygen to your muscles according to the oxygen delivery steps listed above.

Types of Exercise that Improve Cardiorespiratory Fitness

Group I Cardiorespiratory Exercise Activities

> Group I exercise activities require very little skill and provide a constant intensity level. Activities classified as Group I are generally the most ideal for improvement and maintenance of cardiorespiratory fitness. Examples of Group I activities include walking, jogging, running, cycling (on a stationary bicycle), rowing (on a stationary rowing machine), stair climbing (on actual stairs or a machine), and elliptical training (on an elliptical machine).

Group II Cardiorespiratory Exercise Activities

> Group II activities require more skill than Group I activities. Intensity level and energy expenditure will be dependent on the skill level of the individual. Group II activities can be as effective as Group I activities for improving and maintaining cardiorespiratory fitness *if* the person exercising is skilled enough at their chosen activity to maintain the necessary minimum exercise intensity level. Examples of Group II activities include swimming, aerobic dance classes, cycling (on a real bicycle), skating, in-line skating, skipping rope, and nordic skiing.

Group III Cardiorespiratory Exercise Activities

> Group III activities incorporate a large variety of skill requirements and intensity levels.

They are generally more fun than Group I and Group II activities and are good ways to make cardiorespiratory training more enjoyable. Since the intensity levels are less easily controlled for Group III activities, they are more suitable for the maintenance stage, rather than the improvement stage, of cardiorespiratory fitness training. Examples of Group III activities include racquet sports, basketball, and volleyball.

Physical Literacy

The term "physical literacy" may sound intimidating, but it is actually a simple concept.

Physical literacy is merely about developing the fundamental movement skills that all children need, such as running, hopping, throwing, catching and jumping. These movement skills in turn give kids the confidence to participate in different physical activities, sports, and games.

In the same way a child learns to speak by interacting with her parents from an early age, the same is true of learning to move with confidence.

It doesn't require special equipment or training, just a bit of knowledge and the simple and natural desire to give your kid the right building blocks from the start.

The Elements of Physical Literacy

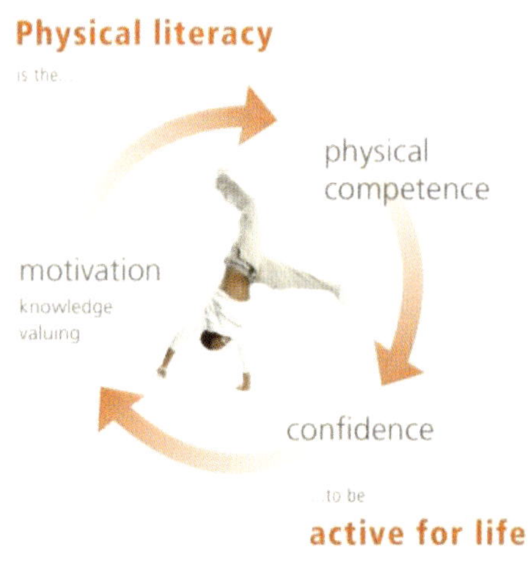

Motivation and Confidence (Affective):

Motivation and confidence refers to an individual's enthusiasm for, enjoyment of, and self-assurance in adopting physical activity as an integral part of life.

Physical Competence (Physical):

Physical competence refers to an individual's ability to develop movement skills and patterns, and the capacity to experience a variety of movement intensities and durations. Enhanced physical competence enables an individual to participate in a wide range of physical activities and settings.

Knowledge and Understanding (Cognitive):

Knowledge and understanding includes the ability to identify and express the essential qualities that influence movement, understand the health benefits of an active lifestyle, and appreciate appropriate safety features associated with physical activity in a variety of settings and physical environments.

Engagement in Physical Activities for Life (Behavioural):

Engagement in physical activities for life refers to an individual taking personal responsibility for physical literacy by freely choosing to be active on a regular basis. This involves prioritizing and sustaining involvement in a range of meaningful and personally challenging activities, as an integral part of one's lifestyle.

References

- Block, Martin (2016). A Teacher's Guide to Adapted Physical Education. Baltimore, Maryland: Paul H. Brookes Publishing Co. pp. 68–74. ISBN 978-1-59857-669-6
- Wang, L., Myers, D., & Yanes, M. (2010). Creating student-centered learning experience through the assistance of high-end technology in physical education. Journal of Instructional Psychology, 37(4), 352–356
- "Physical Education – Jul 18, 1975 – NBC – TV news: Vanderbilt Television News Archive". Tvnews.vanderbilt.edu. 1975-07-18. Retrieved 2015-08-13
- Wilmore J.; Knuttgen H. (2003). "Aerobic Exercise and Endurance Improving Fitness for Health Benefits". The Physician and Sportsmedicine. 31 (5): 45. doi:10.3810/psm.2003.05.367
- Department Of Health And Human Services, United States (1996). "Physical Activity and Health". United States Department of Health. ISBN 9781428927940
- Dobbins, Maureen; Husson, Heather; DeCorby, Kara; LaRocca, Rebecca L (28 February 2013). Cochrane Database of Systematic Reviews. John Wiley & Sons, Ltd. doi:10.1002/14651858.cd007651.pub2
- "American Heart Association Recommendations for Physical Activity in Adults". American Heart Association. 14 December 2017. Retrieved 5 May 2018
- Lumeng, Julie C (2006). "Small-group physical education classes result in important health benefits". The Journal of Pediatrics. 148(3): 418–419. doi:10.1016/j.jpeds.2006.02.025

Chapter 2

Gymnastics and its Types

Gymnastics is a sport or a set of exercises that involves coordination, physical agility, strength, flexibility and endurance. All the major muscle groups such as those of the arms, legs, back, shoulders, chest and the abdomen are stimulated in gymnastics. The topics elaborated in this chapter include acrobatic gymnastics, artistic gymnastics, rhythmic gymnastics, floor gymnastics, etc.

Gymnastics

Gymnastics, the performance of systematic exercises—often with the use of rings, bars, and other apparatus—either as a competitive sport or to improve strength, agility, coordination, and physical conditioning.

Women's Gymnastics

Women's gymnastics is composed of four events -- vault, floor exercise, balance beam, and uneven bars. Each event attempts to challenge the grace, agility, coordination and strength of the gymnast. The balance beam, perhaps the most challenging event, involves the use of balance and agility while performing acrobatic and dance movements on a 4-inch-wide beam. Vault requires great strength as gymnasts explode off the vault to perform flips in the air, while the uneven bars require coordination in order to swing from bar to bar while switching hands and using various transitions. Floor exercise, which is set to music, seems to be a crowd-pleaser, as female gymnasts incorporate elements of acrobatics and dance that showcase their personality. In each event, gymnasts aim to "stick" their landing by taking no extra steps.

Men's Gymnastics

Men's gymnastics includes floor exercise, pommel horse, still rings, high bar, parallel bars, and vault. Each event requires high levels of power and control. The vault, high bar, still rings and parallel bars showcase the male gymnast's strength as he manages to perform swinging, twisting and flipping movements while maintaining balance. The floor exercise and pommel horse highlight precision, coordination, balance and control.

FIG-recognized Disciplines

The following disciplines are governed by FIG.

Artistic Gymnastics

Artistic Gymnastics is usually divided into Men's and Women's Gymnastics. Men compete on six events: Floor Exercise, Pommel Horse, Still Rings, Vault, Parallel Bars, and Horizontal Bar, while women compete on four: Vault, Uneven Bars, Balance Beam, and Floor Exercise. In some countries, women at one time competed on the rings, high bar, and parallel bars (for example, in the 1950s in the USSR).

In 2006, FIG introduced a new points system for Artistic gymnastics in which scores are no longer limited to 10 points. The system is used in the US for elite level competition. Unlike the old code of points, there are two separate scores, an execution score and a difficulty score. In the previous system, the "execution score" was the only score. It was and still is out of 10.00, except for short exercises. During the gymnast's performance, the judges deduct this score only. A fall, on or off the event, is a 1.00 deduction, in elite level gymnastics. The introduction of the difficulty score is a significant change. The gymnast's difficulty score is based on what elements they perform and is subject to change if they do not perform or complete all the skills, or they do not connect a skill meant to be connected to another. Connection bonuses are where deviation happens most common between the intended and actual difficulty scores, as it can be difficult to connect multiple flight elements. It is very hard to connect skills if the first skill is not performed correctly. The new code of points allows the gymnasts to gain higher scores based on the difficulty of the skills they perform as well as their execution. There is no maximum score for difficulty, as it can keep increasing as the difficulty of the skills increase.

Artistic Events for Women

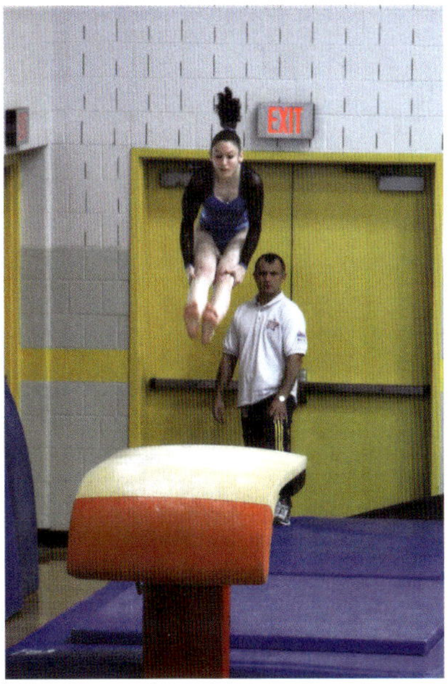

Piked Tsukahara vault.

Vault

In the vaulting events, gymnasts sprint down a 25 metres (82 ft) runway, jump onto a springboard (or perform a roundoff or handspring entry onto a springboard), land momentarily inverted on the hands on the vaulting horse or vaulting table (pre-flight segment), then propel themselves forward or backward off that platform to a two-footed landing (post-flight segment). Every gymnast starts at a different point on the vault runway depending on their height and strength. The post-flight segment may include one or more multiple saltos, somersaults, or twisting movements. A round-off entry vault, called a Yurchenko, is the most common vault in the higher levels in gymnastics. When performing a Yurchenko, gymnasts "round off" so their hands are on the runway while their feet land on the springboard. From the roundoff position, the gymnast travels backwards and executes a back handspring so that the hands land on the vaulting table. The gymnast then blocks off the vaulting platform into various twisting and/or somersaulting combinations. The post-flight segment brings the gymnast to her feet. In the lower levels of gymnastics, the gymnasts do not perform this move. These gymnasts will jump onto the springboard with both feet at the same time and either do a front handspring onto the vault or a roundoff onto the vault.

In 2001, the traditional vaulting horse was replaced with a new apparatus, sometimes known as a tongue, horse or vaulting table. The new apparatus is more stable, wider, and longer than the older vaulting horse, approximately 1 m in length and 1 m in width, giving gymnasts a larger blocking surface. This apparatus is thus considered safer than the vaulting horse used in the past. With the addition of this new, safer vaulting table, gymnasts are attempting more difficult and dangerous vaults.

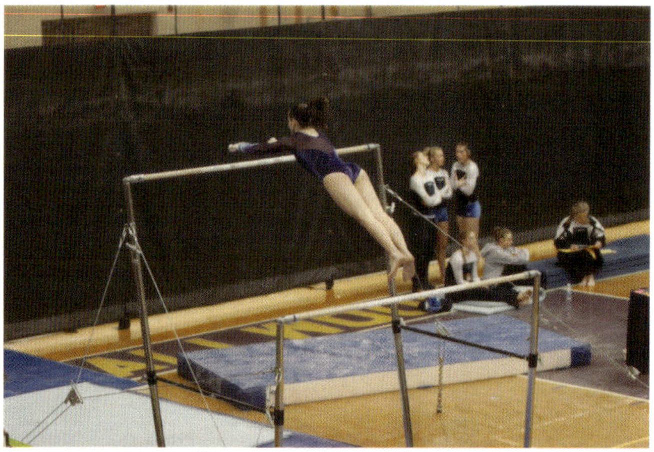

Gymnast on uneven bars.

Uneven Bars

On the uneven bars, the gymnast performs a timed routine on two parallel horizontal bars set at different heights. These bars are made of fiberglass covered in wood laminate, to prevent them from breaking. In the past, bars were made of wood, but the bars were prone to breaking, providing an incentive to switch to newer technologies. The width and height of the bars may be adjusted to the size needed by individual gymnasts. In the past, the uneven parallel bars were closer together. The bars have been moved increasingly further apart, allowing gymnasts to perform swinging, circling, transitional, and release moves that may pass over, under, and between the two bars. At the Elite level, movements must pass through the handstand. Gymnasts often mount the uneven bars using a springboard or a small mat. Chalk ($MgCO_3$) and grips (a leather strip with holes for fingers to protect hands and improve performance) may be used by gymnasts performing this event. The chalk helps take the moisture out of gymnasts' hands to decrease friction and prevent rips (tears to the skin of the hands); dowel grips help gymnasts grip the bar.

Balance Beam

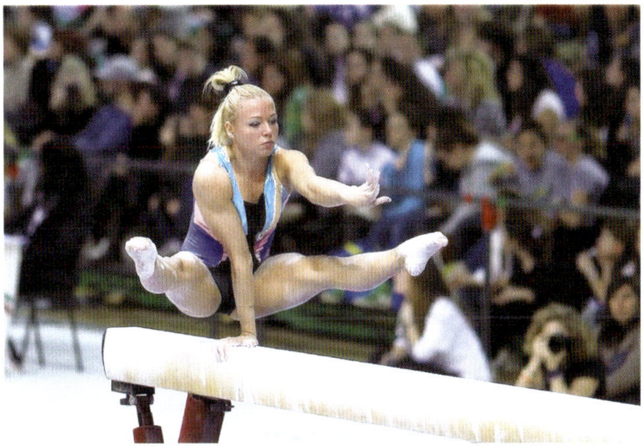

A gymnast performing a one arm press hold during her balance beam mount.

The gymnast performs a choreographed routine of up to 90 seconds in length consisting of leaps, acrobatic skills, somersaults, turns and dance elements on a padded beam. The beam is 125 centimetres (4 ft 1 in) from the ground, 5 metres (16 ft 5 in) long, and 10 centimetres (3.9 in) wide. This stationary object can also be adjusted, to be raised higher or lower. The event requires balance, flexibility, grace, poise, and strength.

Floor

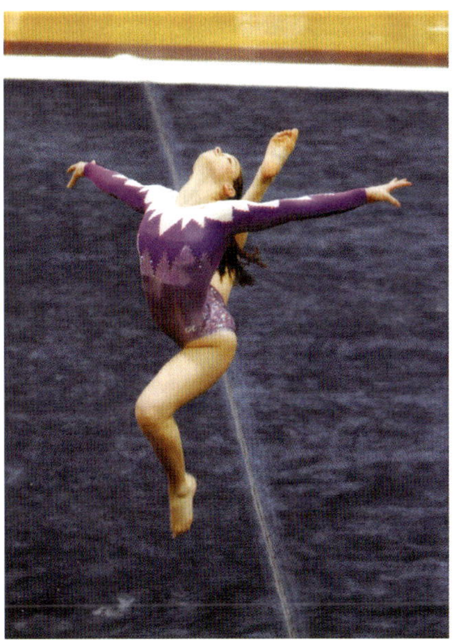

Gymnast doing a stag leap on floor exercise.

The event in gymnastics performed on floor is called floor exercise. The English abbreviation for the event in gymnastics scoring is FX. In the past, the floor exercise event was executed on the bare floor or mats such as wrestling mats. The floor event now occurs on a carpeted 12m × 12m square, usually consisting of hard foam over a layer of plywood, which is supported by springs generally called a "spring" floor. This provides a firm surface that provides extra bounce or spring when compressed, allowing gymnasts to achieve greater height and a softer landing after the composed skill. Gymnasts perform a choreographed routine up to 90 seconds in the floor exercise event; Depending on the level, they may choose their own, or, if known as a "compulsory gymnast," default music must be played. Levels three to six the music is the same for each levels along with the skills within the routine. However, recently, the levels have switched. Now, levels 7-11 are optional levels and they get to have custom routines made. In the optional levels (levels six to ten) there are skill requirements for the routine but the athlete is able to pick her own music without any words. The routine should consist of tumbling passes, series of jumps, leaps, dance elements, acrobatic skills, and turns, or pivots, on one foot. A gymnast can perform up to four tumbling passes that usually includes at least one flight element without hand support. Each level of gymnastics requires the athlete to perform a different number of tumbling passes. In level 7 in the United States, a gymnast is required to do 2–3, and in levels 8–10, at least 3–4 tumbling passes are required.

Artistic Events for Men

Floor

Male gymnasts also perform on a 12meter x 12meter spring floor. A series of tumbling passes are performed to demonstrate flexibility, strength, and balance. Strength skills include circles, scales, and press handstands. Men's floor routines usually have multiple passes that have to total between 60–70 seconds and are performed without music, unlike the women's event. Rules require that male gymnasts touch each corner of the floor at least once during their routine.

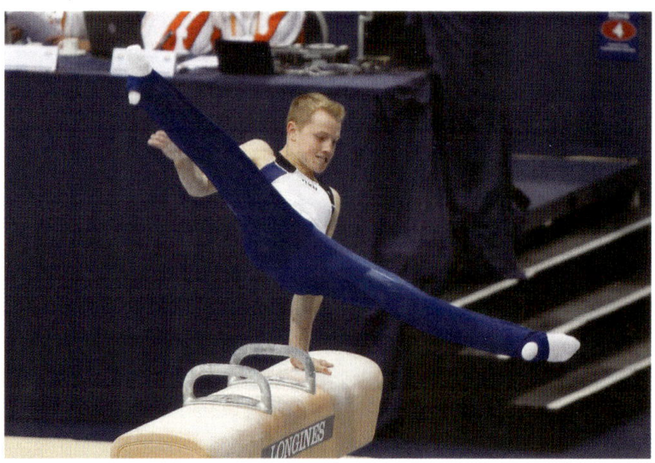

The pommel horse.

Pommel Horse

A typical pommel horse exercise involves both single leg and double leg work. Single leg skills are generally found in the form of scissors, an element often done on the pommels. Double leg work however, is the main staple of this event. The gymnast swings both legs in a circular motion (clockwise or counterclockwise depending on preference) and performs such skills on all parts of the apparatus. To make the exercise more challenging, gymnasts will often include variations on a typical circling skill by turning (moores and spindles) or by straddling their legs (Flares). Routines end when the gymnast performs a dismount, either by swinging his body over the horse, or landing after a handstand variation.

Still Rings

The rings are suspended on wire cable from a point 5.75 meters from the floor. The gymnasts must perform a routine demonstrating balance, strength, power, and dynamic motion while preventing the rings themselves from swinging. At least one static strength move is required, but some gymnasts may include two or three. A routine ends with a dismount.

Vault

Gymnasts sprint down a runway, which is a maximum of 25 meters in length, before hurdling onto a spring board. The gymnast is allowed to choose where they start on the runway. The body position is maintained while "punching" (blocking using only a shoulder movement) the vaulting platform. The gymnast then rotates to a standing position. In advanced gymnastics, multiple twists and somersaults may be added before landing. Successful vaults depend on the speed of the run, the length of the hurdle, the power the gymnast generates from the legs and shoulder girdle, the kinesthetic awareness in the air, how well they stuck the landing and the speed of rotation in the case of more difficult and complex vaults.

Parallel Bars

Men perform on two bars executing a series of swings, balances, and releases that require great strength and coordination. The width between the bars is adjustable dependent upon the actual needs of the gymnasts and usually 2m high.

Horizontal Bar

A 2.8 cm thick steel or fiberglass bar raised 2.5 m above the landing area is all the gymnast has to hold onto as he performs giant swings or *giants* (forward or backward revolutions around the bar in the handstand position), release skills, twists, and changes of direction. By using all of the momentum from giants and then releasing at the proper point, enough height can be achieved for spectacular dismounts, such as a triple-back salto. Leather grips are usually used to help maintain a grip on the bar.

As with women, male gymnasts are also judged on all of their events including their execution, degree of difficulty, and overall presentation skills.

Scoring

A gymnast's score comes from deductions taken from their start value. The start value of a routine is based on the difficulty of the elements the gymnast attempts and whether or not the gymnast meets composition requirements. The composition requirements are different for each apparatus; this score is called the D score. Deductions in execution and artistry are taken from a maximum of 10.0. This score is called the E score. The final score is calculated by taking deductions from the E score, and adding the result to the D score.Since 2007, the scoring system has changed by adding bonus plus the execution and then adding those two together to get the final score.

Landing

In a tumbling pass, dismount or vault, landing is the final phase, following take off and flight This is a critical skill in terms of execution in competition scores, general performance, and injury occurrence. Without the necessary magnitude of energy dissipation during impact, the risk of sustaining injuries during somersaulting increases. These injuries commonly occur at the lower extremities such as: cartilage lesions, ligament tears, and bone bruises/fractures. To avoid such injuries, and to receive a high performance score, proper technique must be used by the gymnast. “The subsequent ground contact or impact landing phase must be achieved using a safe, aesthetic and well-executed double foot landing.” A successful landing in gymnastics is classified as soft, meaning the knee and hip joints are at greater than 63 degrees of flexion.

A higher flight phase results in a higher vertical ground reaction force. Vertical ground reaction force represents external force which the gymnasts have to overcome with their muscle force and affects the gymnasts’ linear and angular momentum. Another important variable that affects linear and angular momentum is time the landing takes. Gymnasts can decrease the impact force by increasing the time taken to perform the landing. Gymnasts can achieve this by increasing hip, knee and ankle amplitude.

Rhythmic Gymnastics

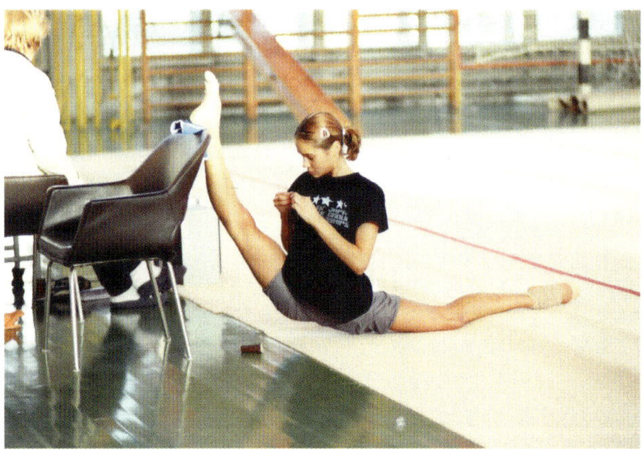

A Russian rhythmic gymnast stretching in her warm-up before practice.

According to FIG rules, only women compete in rhythmic gymnastics. This is a sport that combines elements of ballet, gymnastics, dance, and apparatus manipulation. The sport involves the performance of five separate routines with the use of five apparatus; ball, ribbon, hoop, clubs, rope—on a floor area, with a much greater emphasis on the aesthetic rather than the acrobatic. There are also group routines consisting of 5 gymnasts and 5 apparatuses of their choice. Rhythmic routines are scored out of a possible 30 points; the score for artistry (choreography and music) is averaged with the score for difficulty of the moves and then added to the score for execution.

International competitions are split between Juniors, under sixteen by their year of birth; and Seniors, for women sixteen and over again by their year of birth. Gymnasts in Russia and Europe typically start training at a very young age and those at their peak are typically in their late teens (15–19) or early twenties. The largest events in the sport are the Olympic Games, World Championships, European Championships, World Cup and Grand-Prix Series. The first World Championships were held in 1963 with its first appearance at the Olympics in 1984.

Rhythmic Gymnastics Apparatus

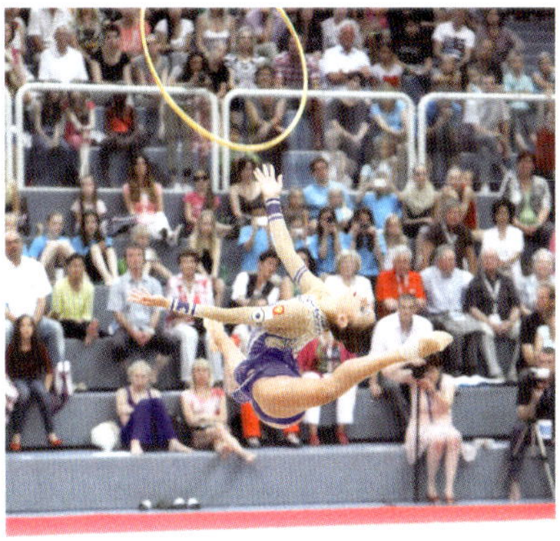
A rhythmic gymnast doing a Split leap in her hoop routine.

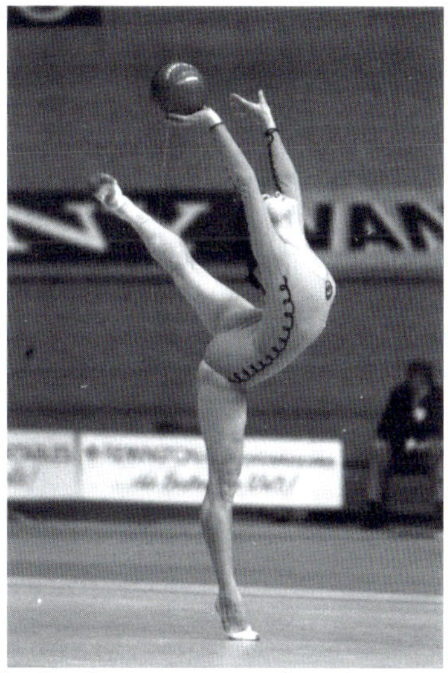
A rhythmic gymnast performing an Attitude balance in her ball apparatus.

Ball: It is made of either rubber or synthetic material (pliable plastic) provided it possesses the same elasticity as rubber. It is from 18 to 20 cm in diameter and must have a minimum weight of 400g. The ball can be of any colour and should rest in the gymnast's hand, not the wrist. Fundamental elements of a ball routine include throwing, bouncing, and rolling. The gymnast must use both hands and work on the whole floor area while showing continuous flowing movement. The ball is to emphasize the gymnast's flowing lines and body difficulty.

Hoop: A hoop is an apparatus in rhythmic gymnastics and may be made of plastic or wood, provided that it retains its shape during the routine. The interior diameter is from 51 to 90 cm, and the hoop must weigh a minimum of 300g. The hoop may be of a natural colour or be partially of fully covered by one or several colours, and it may be covered with adhesive tape either of the same or different colour as the hoop. Fundamental requirements of a hoop routine include rotation around the hand or body and rolling, as well as swings, circles, throws, and passes through and over the hoop. The routines in hoop involves mastery in both apparatus handling and body difficulty like leaps, jumps and pivots.

Ribbon: It is made of satin or another similar material cloth of any colour and may be multi-coloured as well as have designs on it. The ribbon itself must be at least 35g (1 oz), 4–6 cm

(1.6–2.4") in width and for senior category a minimum length of 6m (20') (5m (16.25') for juniors). The ribbon must be in one piece. The end that is attached to the stick is doubled for a maximum length of 1m (3'). This is stitched down both sides. At the top, a very thin reinforcement or rows of machine stitching for a maximum length of 5 cm is authorized. This extremity may end in a strap, or have an eyelet (a small hole, edged with buttonhole stitch or a metal circle), to permit attaching the ribbon. The ribbon is fixed to the stick by means of a supple attachment such as thread, nylon cord, or a series of articulated rings. The attachment has a maximum length of 7 cm (2.8"), not counting the strap or metal ring at the end of the stick where it will be fastened. Compulsory elements for the ribbon include flicks, circles, snakes and spirals, and throws. It requires a high degree of co-ordination to form the spirals and circles as any knots which may accidentally form in the ribbon are penalised. During a ribbon routine, large, smooth and flowing movements are looked for.

Clubs: Multi-piece clubs are the most popular clubs. The club is built along an internal rod, providing a base on which a handle made of polyolefin plastic is wrapped, providing an airspace between it and the internal rod. This airspace provides flex, cushioning impact, making the club softer on the hands. Foam ends and knobs further cushion the club. Multi-piece clubs are made in both a thin European style or larger bodied American style and in various lengths, generally ranging from 19 to 21 inches (480 to 530 mm). The handles and bodies are typically wrapped with decorative plastics and tapes. The skills involved are apparatus mastery and body elements, Clubs are thrown from alternate hands; each passes underneath the other clubs and is caught in the opposite hand to the one from which it was thrown. At its simplest, each club rotates once per throw, the handle moving down and away from the throwing hand at first. However, double and triple spins are frequently performed, allowing the club to be thrown higher for more advanced patterns and to allow tricks such as 360s to be performed underneath.

Trampolining and Tumbling

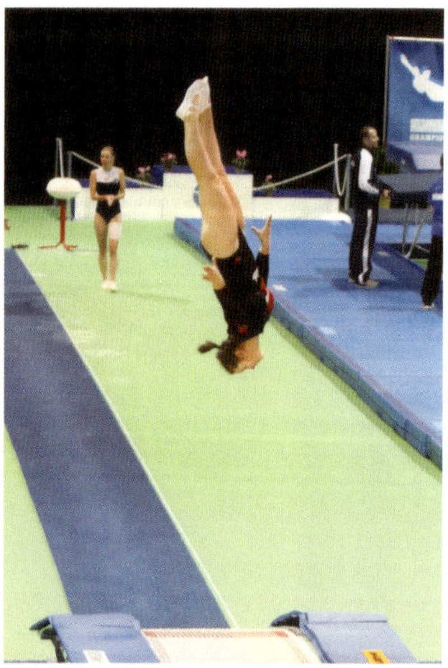

Double mini-trampoline competitor

Trampolining

Trampolining and tumbling consists of four events, individual and synchronized trampoline, double mini trampoline, and tumbling (also known as power tumbling or rod floor). Since 2000, individual trampoline has been included in the Olympic Games. The first World Championships were held in 1964.

Individual Trampoline

Individual routines in trampolining involve a build-up phase during which the gymnast jumps repeatedly to achieve height, followed by a sequence of ten bounces without pause during which the gymnast performs a sequence of aerial skills. Routines are marked out of a maximum score of 10 points. Additional points (with no maximum at the highest levels of competition) can be earned depending on the difficulty of the moves and the length of time taken to complete the ten skills which is an indication of the average height of the jumps. In high level competitions, there are two preliminary routines, one which has only two moves scored for difficulty and one where the athlete is free to perform any routine. This is followed by a final routine which is optional. Some competitions restart the score from zero for the finals, other add the final score to the preliminary results.

Synchronized Trampoline

Synchronized trampoline is similar except that both competitors must perform the routine together and marks are awarded for synchronization as well as the form and difficulty of the moves.

Double-mini Trampoline

Double mini trampoline involves a smaller trampoline with a run-up, two scoring moves are performed per routine. Moves cannot be repeated in the same order on the double-mini during a competition. Skills can be repeated if a skill is competed as a mounter in one routine and a dismount in another. The scores are marked in a similar manner to individual trampoline.

Tumbling

In tumbling, athletes perform an explosive series of flips and twists down a sprung tumbling track. Scoring is similar to trampolining. Tumbling was originally contested as one of the events in Men's Artistic Gymnastics at the 1932 Summer Olympics, and in 1955 and 1959 at the Pan American Games. From 1974 to 1998 it was included as an event for both genders at the Acrobatic Gymnastics World Championships. The event has also been contested since 1976 at the Trampoline World Championships. Since the recognition of Trampoline and Acrobatic Gymnastics as FIG disciplines in 1999, official Tumbling competitions are only allowed as an event in Trampoline gymnastics meets.

Acrobatic Gymnastics

Acrobatic gymnastics (formerly Sport Acrobatics), often referred to as "Acro" if involved with the sport, acrobatic sports or simply sports acro, is a group gymnastic discipline for both men and women. Acrobats in groups of two, three and four perform routines with the heads, hands and feet of their partners. They may, subject to regulations (e.g. no lyrics), pick their own music.

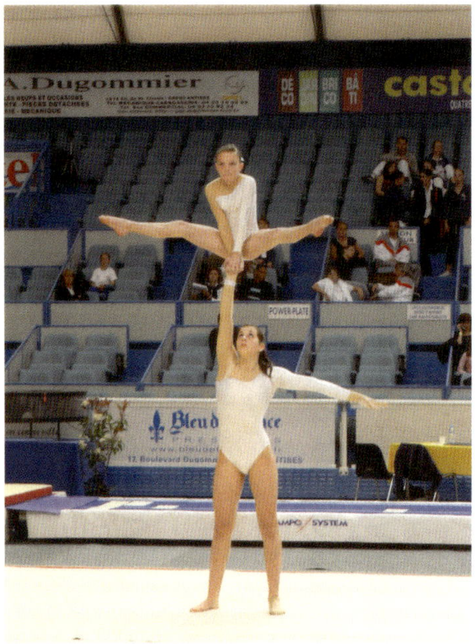

Acrobatic Women's Pair performing a skill.

There are four international age categories: 11-16, 12-18, 13-19, and Senior (15+), which are used in the World Championships and many other events around the world, including European Championships and World Games. All levels require a balance and dynamic routine; 12-18, 13-19, and Seniors are also required to perform a final (combined) routine.

Currently, acrobatic gymnastics is marked out of 30.00 (can be higher at Senior FIG level based on difficulty):

- 10.00 for routine difficulty (valued from the tables of difficulties)
- 10.00 for technical performance (how well the skills are executed)
- 10.00 for artistry (the overall performance of the routine, namely choreography)

The events consist of:

- Women's Pairs
- Mixed Pairs
- Men's Pairs
- Women's Group of 3
- Men's Group of 4

Most competitions require a balance and dynamic routine for each event, though some will do a single mixed event.

The World Championships have been held since 1974.

Aerobic Gymnastics

Aerobic gymnastics (formally Sport Aerobics) involves the performance of routines by individuals, pairs, trios or groups up to 6 people, emphasizing strength, flexibility, and aerobic fitness rather than acrobatic or balance skills. Routines are performed for all individuals on a 7x7m floor and also for 12–14 and 15-17 trios and mixed pairs. From 2009, all senior trios and mixed pairs were required to be on the larger floor (10x10m), all groups also perform on this floor. Routines generally last 60–90 seconds depending on age of participant and routine category. The World Championships have been held since 1995.

The events consist of:

- Individual Women
- Individual Men
- Mixed Pairs
- Trios
- Groups
- Dance
- Step

Parkour

On January 28, 2018 Parkour was given the go ahead to begin development as a FIG sport. The FIG is planning to run World Cup competitions from 2018 onwards and will hold the first Parkour World Championships in 2020.

The events consist of:

- Speedrun
- Freestyle

Other Disciplines

The following disciplines are not currently recognized by the Fédération Internationale de Gymnastique.

Aesthetic Group Gymnastics

Aesthetic Group Gymnastics (AGG) was developed from the Finnish "naisvoimistelu". It differs from Rhythmic Gymnastics in that body movement is large and continuous and teams are larger. Athletes do not use apparatus in international AGG competitions compared to Rhythmic Gymnastics where ball, ribbon, hoop and clubs are used on the floor area. The sport requires physical qualities such as flexibility, balance, speed, strength, coordination and sense of rhythm where movements of the body are emphasized through the flow, expression and aesthetic appeal. A good performance is characterized by uniformity and simultaneity. The competition program consists of versatile and varied body movements, such as body waves, swings, balances, pivots, jumps and leaps, dance steps, and lifts. The International Federation of Aesthetic Group Gymnastics (IFAGG) was established in 2003. The first Aesthetic Group Gymnastics World Championships was held in 2000.

Men's Rhythmic Gymnastics

Men's rhythmic gymnastics is related to both men's artistic gymnastics and wushu martial arts. It emerged in Japan from stick gymnastics. Stick gymnastics has been taught and performed for many years with the aim of improving physical strength and health. Male athletes are judged on some of the same physical abilities and skills as their female counterparts, such as hand/body-eye co-ordination, but tumbling, strength, power, and martial arts skills are the main focus, as opposed to flexibility and dance in women's rhythmic gymnastics. There are a growing number of participants, competing alone and on a team; it is most popular in Asia, especially in Japan where high school and university teams compete fiercely. As of 2002, there were 1000 men's rhythmic gymnasts in Japan.

The technical rules for the Japanese version of men's rhythmic gymnastics came around the 1970s. For individuals, only four types of apparatus are used: the double rings, the stick, the rope, and the clubs. Groups do not use any apparatus. The Japanese version includes tumbling performed on a spring floor. Points are awarded based a 10-point scale that measures the level of difficulty of the tumbling and apparatus handling. On November 27–29, 2003, Japan hosted first edition of the Men's Rhythmic Gymnastics World Championship.

The Events consist of:

- Stick
- Clubs
- Rope
- Double Rings
- Group

TeamGym

TeamGym is a form of competition created by the European Union of Gymnastics, named originally EuroTeam. The first official competition was held in Finland in 1996. TeamGym events consist of three sections: women, men and mixed teams. Athletes compete in three different disciplines: floor, tumbling and trampette. In common for the performance is effective teamwork, good technique in the elements and spectacular acrobatic skills. There is no World Championships however there has been a European Championships held since 2010.

Wheel Gymnastics

Wheel gymnasts do exercises in a large wheel known as the Rhönrad, gymnastics wheel, gym wheel, or German wheel, in the beginning also known as ayro wheel, aero wheel, and Rhon rod.

There are four core categories of exercise: straight line, spiral, vault and cyr wheel. The first World Championships was held in 1995.

Mallakhamba

Mallakhamba is a traditional Indian sport in which a gymnast performs feats and poses in concert with a vertical wooden pole or rope. The word also refers to the pole used in the sport.

Mallakhamba derives from the terms *malla* which denotes a wrestler and *khamba* which means a pole. Mallakhamba can therefore be translated to English as "pole gymnastics". On April 9, 2013, the Indian state of Madhya Pradesh declared mallakhamba as the state sport.

Non-competitive Gymnastics

General gymnastics enables people of all ages and abilities to participate in performance groups of 6 to more than 150 athletes. They perform synchronized, choreographed routines. Troupes may consist of both genders and are not separated into age divisions. The largest general gymnastics exhibition is the quadrennial World Gymnaestrada which was first held in 1939. In 1984 Gymnastics for All was officially recognized first as a Sport Program by the FIG (International Gymnastic Federation), and subsequently by national gymnastic federations worldwide with participants that now number 30 million.

Former Apparatus and Events

Rope (Rhythmic Gymnastics)

This apparatus may be made of hemp or a synthetic material which retains the qualities of lightness and suppleness. Its length is in proportion to the size of the gymnast. The rope should, when held down by the feet, reach both of the gymnasts' armpits. One or two knots at each end are for keeping hold of the rope while doing the routine. At the ends (to the exclusion of all other parts of the rope) an anti-slip material, either coloured or neutral may cover a maximum of 10 cm (3.94 in). The rope must be coloured, either all or partially and may either be of a uniform diameter or be progressively thicker in the center provided that this thickening is of the same material as the rope. The fundamental requirements of a rope routine include leaps and skipping. Other elements include swings, throws, circles, rotations and figures of eight. In 2011, the FIG decided to nullify the use of rope in rhythmic gymnastic competitions.

Rope Climbing

Generally, competitors climbed either a 6m (6.1m = 20 ft in US) or an 8m (7.6m = 25 ft in US), 38 mm diameter (1.5-inch) natural fiber rope for speed, starting from a seated position on the floor and using only the hands and arms. Kicking the legs in a kind of "stride" was normally permitted. Many gymnasts can do this in the straddle or pike position, which eliminates the help generated from the legs though it can be done with legs as well.

Flying Rings

Flying rings was an event similar to still rings, but with the performer executing a series of stunts while swinging. It was a gymnastic event sanctioned by both the NCAA and the AAU until the early 1960s.

Club Swinging

Club Swinging a.k.a. Indian Clubs was an event in Men's Artistic Gymnastics sometimes up until the 1950s. It was similar to the clubs in both Women's and Men's Rhythmic Gymnastics but much simpler with few throws allowed. It was practice. It was competed in the 1904 and 1932 summer Olympic Games.

Other (Men's Artistic)

- Team horizontal bar and parallel bar in the 1896 Summer Olympics
- Team free and Swedish system in the 1912 and 1920 Summer Olympics
- Combined and triathlon in the 1904 Summer Olympics
- Side horse vault in 1924 Summer Olympics
- Tumbling in the 1932 Summer Olympics

Other (Women's Artistic)

- Team exercise at the 1928, 1936, and 1948 Summer Olympics
- Parallel bars at the 1938 World Championships
- Team portable apparatus at the 1952 and 1956 Summer Olympics

Benefits of Gymnastics

Gymnastics is widely renowned as a sport that can improve overall fitness, strength, balance and body control (Harrell, 2003), as well as helping to improve athletic performance in any other sport.

However, what many people don't realise is that extended participation in gymnastics classes also provides many additional cognitive and psychological benefits that will continue to benefit an individual throughout their life. These include:

- Social interaction and discipline;
- Improved mental focus and concentration;
- Education and an understanding of physics;
- Flexibility, balance and co-ordination;
- Numerous health benefits.

Gymnastics and Discipline

Gymnastics provides a unique and valuable social education and experience. It provides an ideal opportunity to learn about teamwork; sportsmanship; fair play and dedication. The time required to master the fundamental skills requires a great amount of patience, dedication, perseverance and planning. Regular gymnastics therefore helps people learn to work hard for objectives that can take years to achieve.

In the modern world of quick-fixes, instant communication and fast food there is a need for young people to develop their character using methods of delayed gratification and gymnastics is a perfect activity for such development.

Gymnastics and Cognitive Functioning

Participation in gymnastics does not only offer physical gains; it is beneficial for improving concentration and mental focus – an important aspect of anyone's life. Studies show that there is a particularly significant relationship between physical activity and cognitive functioning in children (Etnier & Sibley, 2003) and with gymnastics covering such a diverse area, cognitive application is important throughout the entire scope of activities.

From a young age children are encouraged to use play to build upon their understanding of how their body works. The use of gymnastic equipment allows faster development of this process through interaction. Both children and coaches are encouraged to use their imagination, act out situations and develop relationships within the sport. By training the body to perform independently as well as interacting with static equipment, the ability for faster development of spatial awareness and body control is achieved. Gymnastics allows children the chance to think for themselves, to stimulate their imaginations and to solve problems safely.

Children will also experience better hand-eye coordination and improve various communication skills. And as well as taking enjoyment from participation, gymnastics provides a way for young people to test their mettle against themselves and others. Gymnastics can therefore provide opportunities for physical development, character development and education that are hard to find anywhere else .

Gymnastics and Education

Education is perhaps the most important part of gymnastics. When an activity is naturally orchestrated to provide participants with unique and valuable learning experiences, it serves the participants better than any book, television show, or website. As time progresses, noticeable benefits in performance provide individuals with a high level of self-motivation and allow further enjoyment and progression within the sport. This pursuit of success indicates a "healthier" outlook on competition, an improvement in self esteem and an understanding of the importance to function independently and be self-reliant.

One of the most interesting elements of the activities involved in gymnastics is that the gymnast can experience a variety of effects in practice rather than just in theory. For example, physicists discuss the principle of conservation of angular momentum; the gymnast experiences it. The physics teacher may discuss moment of inertia and its relation to angular momentum, but the gymnast can see and feel this while performing skills. The richness of such experiences goes far beyond reading about them in a book. Recently, a National Science Foundation grant has used gymnastics as a means of teaching fundamental physics to students for this very reason.

Gymnastics and Co-Ordination

Flexibility is a big factor in gymnastics. In order to achieve the various positions needed to perform moves, suppleness is of vital importance. Increasing flexibility can also be an effective aid to the reduction of injury, preventing people from forcing a limb to an injurious range of motion. By learning movements and combining them in a routine, the gymnast can attain greater flexibility and greater control of the body.

Gymnastics can also improve co-ordination. Gymnasts do not react with as large a "startle response" to sudden imbalances as non-gymnasts. By applying this conditioning outside the sport, people become better equipped to avoid hazardous situations by quickly identifying them and naturally correcting body alignment when walking, standing or jumping etc. This therefore means that gymnasts can tolerate larger disturbances to their posture because they have become more familiar with these positions.

Gymnastics and Health

Gymnastics moves themselves are designed on a progressive scale to allow further development to make them harder and more intricate. With each level achieved through suitably planned training, participants are able to improve their joint health, maintain muscular development and improve cardiovascular fitness.

Long-term use of weight bearing activities such as gymnastics can also provide a clear benefit in age-related functional decline and bone loss (Uusi-Rasi et al., 2005), helping to reduce the risk of osteoporosis. And because it helps burn fat, a regular workout such as gymnastics also contributes to weight management and in turn, healthy cholesterol levels and blood pressure levels.

Rhythmic Gymnastics

Rhythmic gymnastics, also called modern gymnastics or modern rhythmic gymnastics, the performance of systematic physical exercise with the aid of such hand apparatuses as ropes, hoops, balls, clubs, and ribbons. It is closely related to women's artistic gymnastics—a sport performed on the vaulting horse, uneven parallel bars, balance beam, and floor—and, like synchronized swimming, is allied with dance. The sport dates from the 18th century; and, although some gymnasts participated at the Olympic Games from 1948 to 1956 in individual and group exercises, it was not until the 1984 Olympiad that individual competition became an official competitive event. The 1996 Olympics was the first to include group competition. World championships have been held biannually, in a succession of host cities, since 1963.

An individual routine is performed by one gymnast with one apparatus for 1–11/2 minutes, whereas a group routine is performed by six gymnasts with six pieces of apparatus for 21/2–3 minutes. Both are accompanied by a single musical instrument, usually a piano. The length of the rope used is determined by the height of the individual participant; the plastic or wooden hoop's interior diameter may vary from 80 to 90 cm (32 to 36 inches); the plastic or rubber ball has a diameter of 18 to 20 cm (7 to 8 inches) and must weigh a minimum of 400 grams (14 ounces); a pair of clubs, 40–50 cm (16–20 inches) long, must each weigh a minimum of 150 grams (5.25 ounces); and the ribbon, a satin strip 4 cm (1.6 inches) wide and 7 metres (23 feet) long, is attached to a slender, flexible wooden stick, or cane, that is 50–60 cm (20–24 inches) in length. The apparatus can be of any colour except gold, silver, or bronze.

There are no compulsory elements at the elite and international levels in rhythmic gymnastics, although at least two superior moves (three at the Olympics) and six elements of difficulty are expected to be executed in any one exercise. Artistry—including originality of routine and its execution, gestures and facial expressions, and fluidity of line and movement—counts far more than vigorous acrobatics in scoring points.

Apparatus

The FIG selects which apparatus will be used in competitions; only four out of the five possible apparatuses are sanctioned. Up to 2010, the clubs were not used at the senior level. For 2011, rope was dropped for senior national individual and group competition. In 2011, it was to be dropped for junior national individual competition but returned again in 2015. Rope appeared in junior national group competition in 2011–2012. In 2017, rope appeared in senior group competition.

An individual athlete only manipulates one apparatus at a time. When multiple gymnasts are performing a routine together a maximum of two types of apparatus may be distributed through the group. An athlete can exchange apparatus with a team member at any time through the routine. Therefore, an athlete can manipulate up to two different pieces of apparatus through the duration of the routine.

Rope: It may be made of hemp or a synthetic material which retains the qualities of lightness and suppleness. Its length is in proportion to the size of the gymnast. When the middle of the rope is held down by the feet, both ends should reach the gymnasts' armpits. One or two knots at each end are for keeping hold of the rope while doing the routine. At the ends (to the exclusion of all other parts of the rope) an anti-slip material, either coloured or neutral may cover a maximum of 10.0 cm (3.9 in). The rope must be colored, either all or partially. It may be either of a uniform diameter or be progressively thicker in the center provided that this thickening is of the same material as the rope. The fundamental requirements of a rope routine include leaps and skipping. Other elements include swings, throws, circles, rotations and figures of eight. In 2011, the FIG decided to nullify the use of rope in rhythmic gymnastic competitions.

Hoop: A hoop may be made of plastic or wood, provided that it retains its shape during the routine. The interior diameter is from 51 to 90 cm, and the hoop must weigh a minimum of 300g. The hoop may be of a natural color or be partially or fully covered by one or several colors, and it may be covered with adhesive tape either of the same or different color as the hoop. Fundamental requirements of a hoop routine include rotation around the hand or body and rolling, as well as swings, circles, throws, and passes through and over the hoop. The routines in hoop involves mastery in both apparatus handling and body difficulty like leaps, jumps and pivots.

Ball: It is made of either rubber or synthetic material (pliable plastic) provided it possesses the same elasticity as rubber. It is from 18 to 20 cm in diameter and must have a minimum weight of 400g. The ball can be of any color. The ball should rest in the gymnast's hand and not rest against the wrist or be able to be grasped. Fundamental elements of a ball routine include throwing, bouncing or rolling. The gymnast must use both hands and work on the whole floor area whilst showing continuous flowing movement. The ball is to emphasize the gymnasts flowing lines and body difficulty.

Clubs: Multi-piece clubs are the most popular clubs. The club is built along an internal rod, providing a base on which a handle made of polyolefin plastic is wrapped, providing an airspace between it and the internal rod. This airspace provides flex, cushioning impact, making the club softer on the hands. Foam ends and knobs further cushion the club. Multi-piece clubs are made in both a thin European style or larger bodied American style and in various lengths, generally ranging from 19 to 21 inches (480 to 530 millimetres). The handles and bodies are typically wrapped with decorative plastics and tapes. The skills involved are apparatus mastery and body elements, Clubs are thrown from alternate hands; each passes underneath the other clubs and is caught in the opposite hand to the one from which it was thrown. At its simplest, each club rotates once per throw, the handle moving down and away from the throwing hand at first. However, double and triple spins are frequently performed, allowing the club to be thrown higher for more advanced patterns and to allow tricks such as 360s (channes) to be performed underneath.

Ribbon: It is made of satin or another similar material cloth of any color, it may be multi-colored and have designs on it. The ribbon itself must be at least 35 g (1.2 oz), 4–6 cm (1.6–2.4") in width and have a minimum length of 6m (20') for seniors and 5m (16.25') for juniors. The ribbon must be in one piece. The end that is attached to the stick is doubled for a maximum length of 1m (3'). This is stitched down both sides. At the top, a very thin reinforcement or rows of machine stitching for a maximum length of 5 cm is authorized. This extremity may end in a strap, or have an eyelet (a small hole, edged with buttonhole stitch or a metal circle), to permit attaching the ribbon. The ribbon is fixed to the stick by means of a supple attachment such as thread, nylon cord, or a series of articulated rings. The attachment has a maximum length of 7 cm (2.8"), not counting the strap or metal ring at the end of the stick where it will be fastened. Compulsory elements for the ribbon include flicks, circles, snakes and spirals, and throws. It requires a high degree of co-ordination to form the spirals and circles as any knots which may accidentally form in the ribbon are penalized. During a ribbon routine, large, smooth and flowing movements are looked for. The ribbon may not stop moving or else points are taken off.

Acrobatic Gymnastics

Acrobatic Gymnastics is one of the earliest sports known to man since it's start in ancient Egypt, it has seen tremendous growth in popularity in the last few decades. Acro is a dynamic elegant powerful sport that combines dance and high flying extreme acrobatics.

Engaging choreography and brilliant attire are also a part of the sport. The competitors tell a story with their performances, all while capturing the audience's attention with thrilling tempo and graceful balance skills.

The magnificent performances could hardly be accomplished without cooperative effort and mentoring among partners. There are five events incorporated within the acrobatic gymnastics discipline. The events are women's pair, men's pair, mixed pair, women's group (3 participants), and men's group (4 participants). Each pair/group performs routines featuring gymnastics tumbling skills, partner balances, and tempo skills. Balance skills highlight the athletes' strength and flexibility through pyramids and static positions of the top and middle. Dynamic skills involve somersaulting and twisting with landings on the floor or catches by a bottom partner. Routines are performed on the same 40' x 40' spring floor that the artistic gymnasts use to perform floor routines.

Athletes of varying heights, weights, and body types are needed for acrobatic gymnastics. Smaller, more flexible athletes are needed as tops, while taller and stronger athletes are ideal for base positions.

Benefits of Acrobatic Gymnastics

- Enhances balance, co-ordination and agility
- Develops posture and confident body movement, including the ability to land safely
- Challenges the mind and body to reach new goals
- Builds strength and flexibility for challenge in life
- Is the perfect team based sport for people of all ages and abilities

Acrobatic Gymnastics is a beautiful, dynamic and spectacular sport for both men and women. The sport develops courage, strength, stamina, co-ordination, flexibility, jumping abilities, adroitness etc. Sports acrobatics unites its power and poise, with grace and beauty to create an intriguing sport. Acrobats in groups of two, three and four perform routines with the heads, hands and feet of their partners.

Acrobatic Gymnastics has Five Disciplines

- Women's Pairs involves two females (one base and one top).
- Men's Pairs includes two males (one base and one top).
- Mixed Pairs is comprised of a male (the base) and a female (the top).
- Women's Trios (otherwise known as Women's Groups) has a female base, female middle and female top.
- Men's Fours (also known as Men's Groups) utilises four males (base, middle 1, middle 2 and a top).

Artistic Gymnastics

Artistic Gymnastics allows both male and female gymnasts to participate and compete. Men perform in various events that include vault, pommel horse, still rings, parallel bars, high bar and floor. While women compete in vault, balance beam, uneven bars, and floor exercise. Artistic gymnastics focuses mainly on strength, balance, and agility.

"Artististic gymnastics is divided into two branches: women's artistic gymnastics (WAG) and men's artistic gymnastics (MAG)."

Women's Artistic Gymnastics

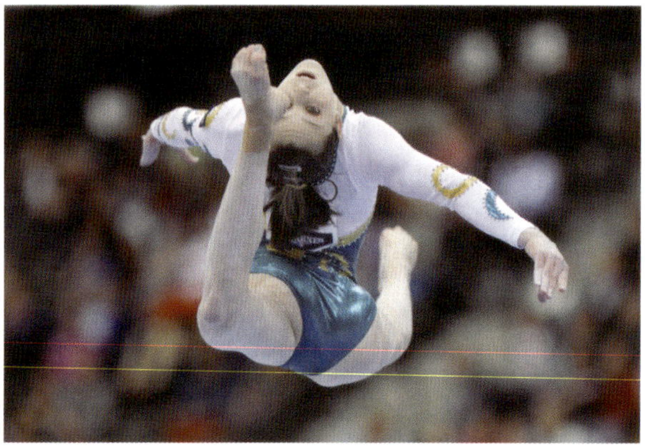

Women's Artisitic Gymnastics is a creative blend of daring and control; powerful yet refined, elegant yet strong. Mastery on the four apparatus requires skills that flip, balance, swing and soar.

- Enhances co-ordination and agility, for body awareness and balance
- Develops posture and confident body movement, including the ability to land safely
- Enhances creativity and builds self-confidence, for sport and life
- Develops strength and flexibility, for life's constant challenges
- Develops healthy minds and bodies for now and later life

Women's Artistic Gymnastics is for women and girls of all ages. Once you've found a club and learnt the basics, you can develop your skills for fun and fitness or challenge yourself further through competitions from local to national, right through to international level.

The four competitive apparatus in Women's Artistic Gymnastics are:

Vault - a 20m sprint to the vaulting table followed by springing onto and off the hands and landing perfectly on the other side. Extra rotations at any point increase the difficulty.

Uneven Bars - requiring strength, precision, rhythm, concentration and courage; the gymnast moves from one bar to the other, alternating grip changes, releases and regrasps, saltos and changes of direction with circular swings.

Beam - balance at its most extreme, adding an extra element to the acrobatic sequences, gymnastic jumps and turns. It is an exercise not only of flexibility, but also of concentration, rhythm and expression.

Floor - a creative combination of expressive dance, daring acrobatics and powerful gymnastics performed to music, where each gymnast communicates her own personality and style.

Men's Artistic Gymnastics

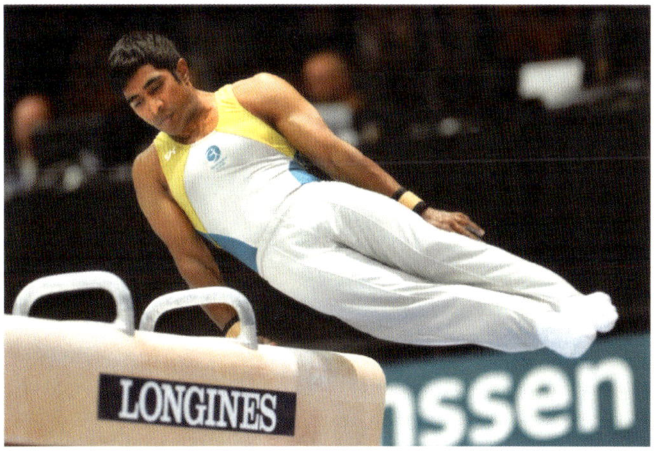

Men's Artistic Gymnastics channels masculine energy to develop power, strength and control. Mastery of the six apparatus requires the skilful combination of flips, balance, stretch, spin and landings.

- Builds strength and prepares the body for the challenges in life
- Enhances co-ordination and agility, allowing the body to move like lightning
- Develops posture and confident body movement, including the ability to land safely
- Challenges the mind and body to reach new goals
- Develops healthy minds and bodies for now and later life

Experience Men's Artistic Gymnastics and feel the exhilaration of being in control as you fly and swing. It is the perfect sport for focus and self-discipline. Once you've found a club, you can develop your skills for fun and fitness or challenge yourself further through competitions from local to national and even international level.

There are six competitive apparatus in Men's Artistic Gymnastics (MAG):

Floor - an exercise in pure acrobatics, alternating between powerful tumbling series and the composure necessary for balance and strength elements.

Pommel Horse - routines mostly involve circles of the legs together and pendulous, scissor swings with the legs split, spectacularly combining these movements while turning and travelling along the horse.

Rings - difficult combination of strength and swinging elements requiring control, strength and balance in the forward and backward swings and strength holds.

Vault - a 25m sprint creates the necessary power to explode from the board before the dynamic push off the table, to generate greater height for rotations and flight before landing on the other side.

Parallel Bars - routines require swinging above and below the bars with acrobatic flight, changes of directions and precise balances, ending in a dramatic dismount off the side or the end of the bars.

Horizontal Bar - a spectacular apparatus, largely due to the combination and variation of giant swings, acrobatic releases and re-grasp flight elements. The high dismounts from the bar allows the gymnast to show his acrobatic talents and landing prowess.

Tumbling

Tumbling is one of the competitive athletic sports incorporated under the broader umbrella of gymnastics. Usually referred to as "trampoline and tumbling," this sport joins those of artistic gymnastics, rhythmic gymnastics and acrobatic gymnastics.

Tumbling is a form of acrobatic activity that involves flips, jumps, rolls, somersaults and handsprings linked together into performance routines and usually performed on a padded floor and choreographed to music. In many ways, a tumbling routine is similar to the floor exercise in gymnastics, although it does not include as many elements of formal dance. Unlike the other elements of gymnastics, tumbling uses no special equipment such as a vault or pommel horse. Tumbling passes may also be used in cheer or dance routines.

Power Tumbling blends the most exciting aspects of an Artistic Gymnastics floor exercise with the dynamics of Trampoline skills. Tumblers perform on a specialized tumbling strip, which is 26 metres long and 1.5 metres wide. The strip is an elevated floor sprung with horizontal fibreglass rods concealed beneath a carpeted layer of foam. The innovation of this specialized 'floor' has raised the level of the sport to new heights. It provides the athletes with an extremely explosive 'launching pad', which can propel the most talented athletes high into the air allowing them to perform combinations of consecutive aerial skills at levels of difficulty not normally seen in Artistic Gymnastics. In competition the athletes perform tumbling lines (connected tumbling skills) called 'passes'. These passes consist of eight acrobatic elements judged on their degree of difficulty and execution – which includes the evaluation of speed, technique, height and maintenance of tempo throughout the entire 8 element pass.

Benefits of Tumbling Classes

Grow Strong Bones

Any weight-bearing activity like tumbling will help your child develop strong, healthy bones. By developing tough bones at a young age, your child will be less at risk for osteoporosis and other bone diseases when they get older.

Reduces Depression

Several forms of exercise have been linked to reducing depression, and tumbling and other gymnastics classes are no exception. By increasing endorphin production, tumbling can help reduce stress, anxiety, and sleep issues.

Improves Self-Confidence

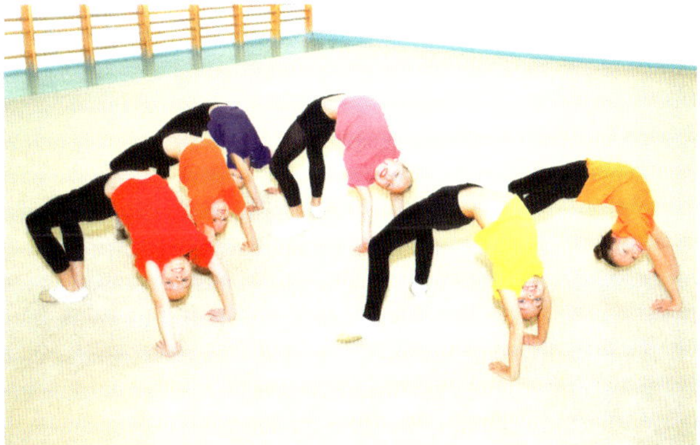

Often, gymnasts will learn not to be too critical of themselves before other kids their age, as performing a tumbling routine for a competition will allow them to develop the skills to analyze their performance as a judge would. This ability will often be applied to other areas of your child's life, and you will find that they have a high self-esteem.

Promotes Healthy Cognitive Function

Tumbling classes can be considered an intense physical activity depending on the age and skill level of the students. As your child advances in their skill level, they'll be asserting more of their energy, which has been linked to improved cognitive function. Gymnastics has been shown to result in higher academic performances and aid in the development of your child's reasoning skills, language communication, memory, learning, and attention span.

Floor

Floor exercise, gymnastics event in which movements are performed on the floor in an area 12 metres (40 feet) square. This area is covered by some type of cloth or mat, usually with some cushioning. No other apparatus is used. Men's routines are 50 to 70 seconds in duration. The type of exercise required is a series of movements combining elements of flexibility, strength, jumps, holding of poses, and balance, as well as other maneuvers. The whole routine must be performed with rhythm and harmony, and the gymnast must move in different directions, using a major portion of the allotted area.

The exercise usually starts and finishes with a series of tumbling movements, such as a handspring or a cartwheel with a half-turn (roundoff), continuing with handsprings and somersaults (in the air), either backward or forward. Between start and finish, balances are held on one leg, handstands are achieved by placing the hands on the floor and kicking to a standing position, and movements resembling ballet, tumbling movements, and jumps are interposed.

The women's event is similar to the men's, except that it is performed to music and lasts 70 to 90 seconds. The floor exercise was introduced as an individual Olympic medal sport for men in 1936 and for women in 1952.

The floor exercise is both a women's artistic gymnastics and men's artistic gymnastics event.

It's the fourth and last of the women's apparatus, competed after vault, uneven bars and balance beam in Olympic order. Men compete on the floor first when performing in Olympic order (floor, pommel horse, rings, vault, parallel bars and high bar).

The Floor Mat

The floor exercise is a square, about 40 feet long by 40 feet wide. It's usually made of foam and springs and covered with carpeting.

Types of Floor Skills

Women perform both tumbling and dance skills on floor, while men do tumbling and occasional strength moves, or flairs and circles.

Dance skills are often similar to the ones shown on beam and include leaps, jumps and turns.

Men and women usually do four or five tumbling passes in a routine, and the passes often contain multiple flips and twists.

Some examples of difficult tumbling skills include the double-twisting double back done in a tucked or layout position; a back three and a half twist; and Arabian double pikes or double layouts.

There are also combination passes, in which a gymnast performs one or more rebounding skills right in a row, and roll-out skills (at 0:10). Women are prohibited from doing roll-out skills, and there are safety concerns with this type of move.

Men are required to do a strength move, which often looks like a move similar to one done on rings. The gymnast will hold a position for two seconds before moving on to the next skill. Sometimes, male gymnasts will do circles or flairs similar to those done on the pommel horse.

The Top Floor Workers

The Women

American Alexandra Raisman won the gold on floor at the 2012 games and did some of the most difficult tumbling ever done by a woman.

Simone Biles, world all-around and floor champion in 2013 and 2014, also did some ultra-difficult skills, including a double layout, half twist, incidentally called the Biles.

In the women's Code of Points, tumbling has become more emphasized than dance and artistry, so you'll see current floor routines with much more tumbling than choreography.

Russian Ksenia Afanasyeva won the 2011 world title on floor and is a stronger dancer than many top floor workers.

Other top floor workers have included Romanian Catalina Ponor (2004 Olympic gold medalist and 2012 silver medalist on floor); Lauren Mitchell (2010 floor world champ and 2009 runner-up); and Sandra Izbasa (2008 Olympic gold medalist on floor).

Another highly decorated American on floor is Dominique Dawes, a four-time national champion on the event and the 1996 Olympic bronze medalist. Dawes was well-known for her unique back-to-back tumbling passes to start her routine.

Nellie Kim, who served as president of the FIG (International Gymnastics Federation) Women's Technical Committee, won two Olympic golds on floor: in 1976 and in 1980 (tied with Nadia Comaneci).

The Men

On the men's side, China's Zou Kai won an Olympic gold in both 2008 and 2012, with very difficult tumbling that sometimes exhibits poor form.

Japanese gymnast Kenzo Shirai won floor at 2013 worlds with more twists than anyone had ever done before — including a quad twist at the end.

Olympic all-around champion Kohei Uchimura won the 2012 Olympic silver medal on floor and was the 2011 world champ with a different strategy: slightly less difficult tumbling, but impeccable form.

Jake Dalton and Steven Legendre have been two other top American gymnasts on the floor. Dalton won a silver at the 2013 worlds, while Legendre was fifth at both the 2011 and 2013 worlds. Peter Kormann, who won a bronze in 1976, became the first American man to have medaled on the floor at the Olympics.

A Floor Routine

Gymnasts must use the entire floor mat during their routine, but cannot step off the floor mat at any time or a deduction is taken.

A floor routine lasts up to 90 seconds. Women perform to music of their choice, while men perform without music.

References

- Loken, Newton C.; Willoughby, Robert J. (1977). The Complete Book of Gymnastics (3rd ed.). Englewood Cliffs, NJ: Prentice-Hall, Inc. ISBN 0-13-157172-9
- Yeow, C., Lee, P., & Goh, J. (2009). Effect of landing height on frontal plane kinematics, kinetics and energy dissipation at lower extremity joints. Journal of Biomechanics , 1967-1973

- Wolf, Megan R.; Avery, Daniel; Wolf, Jennifer Moriatis (February 2017). "Upper Extremity Injuries in Gymnasts". Hand Clinics. 33 (1): 187–197. doi:10.1016/j.hcl.2016.08.010. ISSN 1558-1969. PMID 27886834
- Otake, Tomoko (2013-08-17). "Image-flip for male rhythmic gymnasts". The Japan Times Online. ISSN 0447-5763. Retrieved 2017-07-12
- Goodbody, John (1982). The Illustrated History of Gymnastics. London: Stanley Paul & Co. ISBN 0-09-143350-9
- "WAG Code of Points 2009–2012". FIG. p. 29. Archived from the original (PDF) on 2011-12-19. Retrieved 2009-10-02
- Feeley, Brian T.; Agel, Julie; LaPrade, Robert F. (January 2016). "When Is It Too Early for Single Sport Specialization?". The American Journal of Sports Medicine. 44 (1): 234–241. doi:10.1177/0363546515576899. ISSN 1552-3365. PMID 25825379

Chapter 3

Aerobics: Cardiovascular Exercise

Aerobics is a form of physical activity, which combines strength training with rhythmic aerobic exercise with the objective of augmenting flexibility, cardio-vascular fitness and muscular strength. The diverse forms of aerobic exercise, such as indoor aerobic exercises and outdoor aerobic exercises have been thoroughly discussed in this chapter.

Whether you call it aerobic or cardiovascular or endurance exercise, you're probably talking about the same thing: getting your heart pumping and oxygenated blood flowing, with the goal of improving your cardiorespiratory health. But it benefits more than just your heart.

The technical definition of aerobic exercise is "any form of exercise or activity that uses the aerobic metabolism — meaning oxygen is heavily involved in the cellular reactions that provide the body with the energy necessary to perform activity,".

That means aerobic exercise makes the heart more efficient and capable of moving more oxygen-carrying blood with every beat. The lungs adapt to be able to take in more oxygen, and the muscles become equipped to use more oxygen.

Another way to think about aerobic exercise or "cardio" is that it's the type of workout where your heart rate and breathing increase.

Mechanism of Aerobic Exercise

Mechanisms of aerobic exercise: oxygen transport and consumption, the role of the heart and the muscles, the proven benefits of aerobic exercise, how much you need to do to reap the benefits, and more.

It all starts with breathing. The average healthy adult inhales and exhales about 7 to 8 liters of air per minute. Once you fill your lungs, the oxygen in the air (air contains approximately 20% oxygen) is filtered through small branches of tubes (called bronchioles) until it reaches the alveoli. The alveoli are microscopic sacs where oxygen diffuses (enters) into the blood. From there, it's a beeline direct to the heart.

The heart has four chambers that fill with blood and pump blood (two atria and two ventricles) and some very active coronary arteries. Because of all this action, the heart needs a fresh supply of oxygen, and as you just learned, the lungs provide it. Once the heart uses what it needs, it pumps the blood, the oxygen, and other nutrients out through the large left ventricle and through the circulatory system to all the organs, muscles, and tissues that need it.

Your heart beats approximately 60-80 times per minute at rest, 100,000 times a day, more than 30 million times per year, and about 2.5 billion times in a 70-year lifetime! Every beat of your heart sends a volume of blood (called stroke volume -- more about that later), along with oxygen and many other life-sustaining nutrients, circulating through your body. The average healthy adult heart pumps about 5 liters of blood per minute.

All that oxygen being pumped by the blood is important. You may be familiar with the term "oxygen consumption." In science, it's labeled VO_2, or volume of oxygen consumed. It's the amount of oxygen the muscles extract, or consume from the blood, and it's expressed as ml/kg/minute (milliliters per kilogram of body weight). Muscles are like engines that run on fuel (just like an automobile that runs on fuel); only our muscles use fat and carbohydrates instead of gasoline. Oxygen is a key player because, once inside the muscle, it's used to burn fat and carbohydrate for fuel to keep our engines running. The more efficient our muscles are at consuming oxygen, the more fuel we can burn, the more fit we are, and the longer we can exercise.

Health Benefits of Aerobic Exercise

Cancer Prevention

Colon cancer. Research is clear that physically active men and women have about a 30%-40% reduction in the risk of developing colon cancer compared with inactive individuals. It appears that 30-60 minutes per day of moderate- to vigorous-intensity physical activity is needed to decrease the risk, and there is a dose-response relationship, which means that the risk declines the more active you are. Breast cancer. There is reasonably clear evidence that physically active women have a greater reduction in risk compared with inactive women. Like colon cancer, it appears that 75 to 150 minutes per day of moderate- to vigorous-intensity physical activity is needed to decrease the risk, and it is likely that there is a dose-response relationship as well. Prostate cancer. Research is inconsistent regarding whether physical activity plays any role in the prevention of this cancer. Lung cancer. There are relatively few studies on physical activity and lung cancer prevention. The available data suggest that physically active individuals have a lower risk of lung cancer; however, it is difficult to completely account for the risks of active and passive cigarette smoking as well as radon exposure. Other cancers. There is little information on the role of physical activity in preventing other cancers.

Cancer Treatment

There's some good news for people undergoing cancer treatment. In one study, aerobic exercise performed five days per week for 30-35 minutes for six weeks at 80% of maximal heart rate reduced fatigue in women being treated for cancer. In another study, 10 weeks of aerobic exercise at 60% of maximum heart rate for 30-40 minutes, four days per week, reduced depression and anxiety in female cancer patients. Aerobic exercise isn't a panacea when it comes to cancer, but evidence suggests that it certainly can help.

Osteoporosis

Osteoporosis is a disease characterized by low bone density, which can lead to an increased risk of fracture. The good news is that exercise may increase bone density or at least slow the rate of decrease in both men and women. It may not work for everyone, and the precise amount and type of exercise necessary to accrue benefits is unknown, but there is evidence that it can help. In children there is good news, too. It seems that active children have greater bone density than sedentary children and that this may help prevent fractures later in life.

Depression

Most of us who exercise regularly understand that exercise can elevate our mood. There have been a number of studies investigating the effects of exercise on depression. In one of the most recent studies, it was shown that three to five days per week for 12 weeks of biking or treadmill for approximately 30 minutes per workout reduced scores on a depression questionnaire by 47%. It's not a substitute for therapy in a depression that causes someone to be unable to function (in which case medication and/or psychotherapy may be necessary), but for milder forms of depression, the evidence is persuasive that it can help.

Diabetes

No study has been more conclusive about the role of lifestyle changes (diet and exercise) in preventing diabetes than the Diabetes Prevention Program. It was a study of more than 3,000 individuals at high risk for diabetes who lost 12-15 pounds and walked 150 minutes per week (five 30-minute walks per day) for three years. They reduced their risk of diabetes by 58%. That's significant considering there are 1 million new cases of diabetes diagnosed each year. Aerobic exercise can also improve insulin resistance. Insulin resistance is a condition in which the body doesn't use insulin properly, and this condition can occur in individuals who do and do not have diabetes. Insulin is a hormone that helps the cells in the body convert glucose (sugar) to energy. Many studies have shown the positive effects of exercise on insulin resistance. In one, 28 obese postmenopausal women with type 2 diabetes did aerobic exercise for 16 weeks, three times per week, for 45-60 minutes, and their insulin sensitivity improved by 20%.

Cardiovascular Disease

The list of studies that show that aerobic exercise prevents or reduces the occurrence of cardiovascular disease is so long that it would take this entire article and probably five others just like it to review all of the research. One of the most important is one of the earliest. In a study of more than 13,000 men and women, it was shown that the least fit individuals had much higher rates of cardiovascular disease than fit individuals -- in some cases, the risk was twice as high. Aerobic exercise works in many ways to prevent heart disease; two of the most important are by reducing blood pressure and allowing blood vessels to be more compliant (more compliant means that they become less stiff and it's less likely for fat to accumulate and clog up the vessels). Results like these have been proven over and over again.

Obesity and Weight Control

Aerobic exercise is believed by many scientists to be the single best predictor of weight maintenance. You can lose weight without exercise by reducing your caloric intake enough so that you burn more calories than you consume, but it takes a regular dose of exercise to keep your weight off. How much is not clear, but somewhere between 30 and 40 minutes of vigorous exercise several times per week, to 45 to 75 minutes of moderate intensity exercise five or more days per week is probably about right.

There are numerous performance benefits:

- Increased storage of energy molecules such as fats and carbohydrates within the muscles, allowing for increased endurance
- Neovascularization of the muscle sarcomeres to increase blood flow through the muscles
- Increasing speed at which aerobic metabolism is activated within muscles, allowing a greater portion of energy for intense exercise to be generated aerobically
- Improving the ability of muscles to use fats during exercise, preserving intramuscular glycogen
- Enhancing the speed at which muscles recover from high intensity exercise
- Neurobiological effects: improvements in brain structural connections and increased gray matter density, new neuron growth, improved cognitive function (cognitive control and various forms of memory), and improvement or maintenance of mental health

Some drawbacks of aerobic exercise include:

- Overuse injuries because of repetitive, high-impact exercise such as distance running.
- Is not an effective approach to building muscle.
- Only effective for fat loss when used consistently.

Both the health benefits and the performance benefits, or "training effect", require a minimum duration and frequency of exercise. Most authorities suggest at least twenty minutes performed at least three times per week.

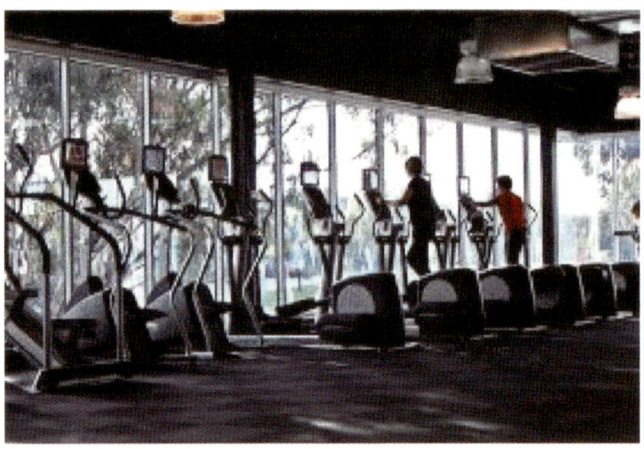

Aerobic workout.

Cooper himself defines aerobic exercise as the ability to utilise the maximum amount of oxygen during exhaustive work. Cooper describes some of the major health benefits of aerobic exercise, such as gaining more efficient lungs by maximising breathing capacity, thereby increasing ability to ventilate more air in a shorter period of time. As breathing capacity increases, one is able to extract oxygen more quickly into the blood stream, increasing elimination of carbon dioxide. With aerobic exercise the heart becomes more efficient at functioning, and blood volume, hemoglobin and red blood cells increase, enhancing the ability of the body to transport oxygen from the lungs into the blood and muscles. Metabolism will change and enable consumption of more calories without putting on weight. Aerobic exercise can delay osteoporosis as there is an increase in muscle mass, a loss of fat and an increase in bone density. With these variables increasing, there is a decrease in likelihood of diabetes as muscles use sugars better than fat. One of the major benefits of aerobic exercise is that body weight may decrease slowly; it will only decrease at a rapid pace if there is a calorie restriction, therefore reducing obesity rates.

Aerobic Capacity

Aerobic capacity describes the functional capacity of the cardiorespiratory system, (the heart, lungs and blood vessels). Aerobic capacity refers to the maximum amount of oxygen consumed by the body during intense exercises, in a given time frame. It is a function both of cardiorespiratory performance and the maximum ability to remove and utilize oxygen from circulating blood. To measure maximal aerobic capacity, an exercise physiologist or physician will perform a VO_2 max test, in which a subject will undergo progressively more strenuous exercise on a treadmill, from an easy walk through to exhaustion. The individual is typically connected to a respirometer to measure oxygen consumption, and the speed is increased incrementally over a fixed duration of time. The higher the measured cardiorespiratory endurance level, the more oxygen has been transported to and used by exercising muscles, and the higher the level of intensity at which the individual can exercise. More simply put, the higher the aerobic capacity, the higher the level of aerobic fitness. The Cooper and multi-stage fitness tests can also be used to assess functional aerobic capacity for particular jobs or activities.

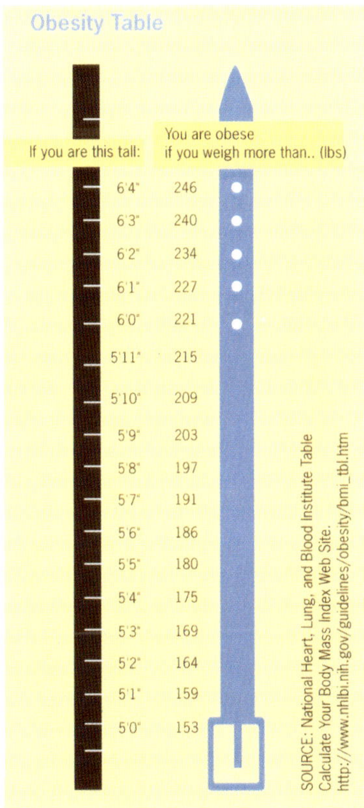

Obesity table.

The degree to which aerobic capacity can be improved by exercise varies very widely in the human population: while the average response to training is an approximately 17% increase in VO_2max, in any population there are "high responders" who may as much as double their capacity, and "low responders" who will see little or no benefit from training. Studies indicate that approximately 10% of otherwise healthy individuals cannot improve their aerobic capacity with exercise at all. The degree of an individual's responsiveness is highly heritable, suggesting that this trait is genetically determined.

Aerobic exercise and obesity

Obesity in Australia is becoming a huge issue, with one in four Australians being overweight. Obesity can be deadly as it increases the risk of coronary heart disease, type 2 diabetes and stroke. In Australia it is proven that nearly 40% of males and 60% of females do not do enough physical activity a day. Introducing aerobic exercise to a daily routine would benefit the body and reduce the risk of cardiovascular disease. The Australian Heart Foundation guidelines outline that exercise to reduce fat should involve continuous moderate aerobic exercise. Continuous moderate exercise is easily accessible and should be performed for at least 30 minutes five times a week. This will reduce obesity by 19% versus no activity at all.

Alternatives

Higher intensity exercise, such as High-intensity interval training (HIIT), increases the resting metabolic rate (RMR) in the 24 hours following high intensity exercise, ultimately burning more calories than lower intensity exercise; low intensity exercise burns more calories during the exercise, due to the increased duration, but fewer afterwards.

"Simple" Aerobic Training

The simplest method of starting is just that, simple. Select the number of minutes you'd like to walk for (let's say 20 minutes for your first walk) and head out the door or step on the treadmill and go for it. Remember that to make it aerobic you want to walk at a pace that leaves you feeling "warm and slightly out of breath" and one that you can sustain for the time that you planned. In this case, set your sights on completing 20 minutes and pace yourself to do it. If you start too quickly, then you may poop out too soon. It's not important how fast you do it; it's just important that you attempt to complete the time. If you find 20 minutes is too ambitious, then start with less.

Five-out, Five-back Training Plan

Interval Training

Interval training is more intense than simple aerobic training. It's a very effective way to increase your fitness level (remember stroke volume and mitochondria activity!), but it's tough, and so it is recommended holding off until you build up to 20-30 minutes of aerobic exercise. The idea to intervals is to set up work to active-rest ratios (work:active-rest), and as you get more fit, decrease the active-rest interval and increase the work interval. The work interval of the ratio is a speed that is faster than what you usually do, and the active-rest interval is your usual speed. To do it, you start at your usual speed for five to eight minutes, then increase the speed to the work interval for one to three minutes, then slow down to your usual speed for a few minutes to catch your breath (this is the active-rest interval), and then you repeat the cycling for the duration of your workout.

Heart Rate Training

You can get more specific with your aerobic interval training and use heart rate since it's an excellent indication of how hard you are working. Let's use jogging on a treadmill as the aerobic activity in this example. For example, if your heart rate is at 70% of your predicted maximum when you jog at 6 mph, then start at that speed and either increase the speed or elevation so that your heart rate increases to 85% or even 90% for one minute, then back to your usual jogging speed for three minutes to elicit a heart rate of 70%. Start with a 1:3 work:active-rest ratio. That's a good starting point, and as you increase the work intervals and decrease the active-rest ratios like in the examples above, you'll notice that your conditioning improves so that your heart rate will be lower at the higher speeds.

Increasing Duration and Intensity

The general rule for increasing aerobic activity is 10% per week. Interestingly, there's no evidence to suggest that a 10% increase is the safest and most effective amount of time to increase, but that's the rule of thumb and it seems to work pretty well. So, if you're walking for 20 minutes then the next increase ought to be two minutes for the following week. The bottom line though is to listen to your body. If you find that increasing by 10% is very easy, then go ahead and try a little more. But if you find that you are tired for hours after your workout, or chronically sore or achy from your workouts, then you know you need to cut back to 10% increases.

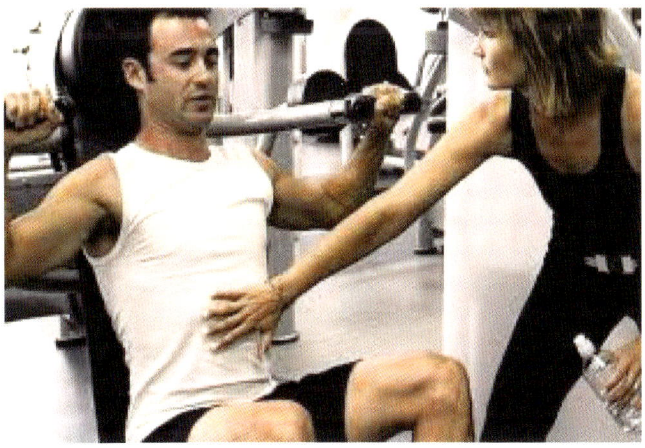

Aerobic Equipment Involved in:

Rowers, treadmills, bikes, and cross-country skiers are all effective if you use them. There is some suggestion that some individuals are more inclined to exercise at home with equipment than at the gym or a class. The activity you choose is a personal choice and it varies for everyone, and so you need to experiment until you find what works best for you. Some individuals prefer to go to the gym while others are perfectly content to work out at home on their own equipment.

Indoor Aerobic Exercises

Indoor Rower

An indoor rower (or rowing machine) is an exercise machine that simulates rowing a watercraft. Indoor rowing is an all-around excellent exercise. First of all, it's a highly effective full-body exercise, but it's also a low-impact workout.

- Full-body exercise – Indoor rowing requires effort from both your upper and lower body. With a lot of major muscle groups in use this is a tough workout. But you can pace yourself, such that this exercise will work for anyone – from novice to athlete.
- Calorie burning efficiency – because it involves your whole body – you can burn a lot of calories – up to 377 in a 30-minute workout. This means efficiency – spend less time working out.
- Low-impact – Indoor rowing involves no jarring impacts to the joints, and doesn't require extreme mobility. For these reasons, this is an excellent cardiovascular and endurance workout for midlifers. It's also great for people who aren't quite ready for weight bearing exercise. And while it can cause some low back strain – using the right form can prevent this.
- Serious aerobic workout – This is a great cardiovascular exercise, it gets your heart pumping and you'll be breathing hard. Oxygen uptake will be through the roof.
- Space efficiency – With the right machine, it takes a minimum of space – which means you can work out year-round, indoors – and away from the heat or the cold.

Design Pattern

All rowing-machine designs consist of an energy damper or braking mechanism connected to a chain, strap, belt and/or handle. Footrests are attached to the same mounting as the energy damper. Most include a rail which either the seat or the mechanism slide upon. Different machines have a variety of layouts and damping mechanisms, each of which have certain advantages and disadvantages.

Currently available ergometer (flywheel-type) rowing machines use a spring or elastic cord to take up the pull chain/strap and return the handle. Advances in elastic cord and spring technology have contributed to the longevity and reliability of this strategy, but it still has disadvantages. With time and usage, an elastic element loses its strength and elasticity. Occasionally it will require adjustment, and eventually it will no longer take up the chain with sufficient vigour, and will need to be replaced. The resilience of an elastic cord is also directly proportional to temperature. In an unheated space in a cold climate, an elastic cord equipped rowing ergometer is unusable because the chain take-up is too sluggish. Thus, as the result of several factors, the force required to stretch the elastic cord is a variable, not a constant. This is of little consequence if the exercise device is used for general fitness, but it is an unacknowledged problem, the "dirty little secret", of indoor rowing competitions. The electronic monitor only measures the user input to the flywheel. It does not measure the energy expenditure to stretch the elastic cord. A claim of a "level playing field" cannot be made when a resistance variable exists (that of the elastic cord) which is not measured or monitored in any way.

In the patent record, means are disclosed whereby the chain/cable take-up and handle return are accomplished without the use of a spring or elastic cord, thereby avoiding the stated disadvantages and defects of this broadly used method. One example is the Gjessing-Nilson device described above. Partially discernable in the thumbnail photo, it utilizes a cable wrapped around a helical pulley on the flywheel shaft, the ends of this cable being connected to opposite ends of a long pole to which a handle is fixed. The obvious disadvantage of this system is the forward space requirement to accommodate the extension of the handle pole at the "catch" portion of the stroke. The advantage is that, except for small transmission losses, all of the user's energy output is imparted to the flywheel, where it can be accurately measured, not split between the flywheel and an elastic cord of variable, unmeasured resistance. If a similar system were installed on all rowing ergometers used in indoor rowing competitions, consistency between machines would be guaranteed because the variability factor of elastic cord resistance would be eliminated, and this would therefore ensure that the monitor displayed actual user energy input.

In a 1988 US patent, Elliot Tarlow discloses another non-elastic chain/cable take-up and handle return strategy. Described and depicted is a continuous chain/cable loop that passes around the flywheel sprocket and around and between fixed pulleys and sprockets positioned fore and aft on the device. The handle is secured in the middle of the exposed upper horizontal section of the chain/cable loop. Although somewhat lacking in aesthetics, the Tarlow device does eliminate the stated disadvantages and defects of the ubiquitous elastic cord handle return. Tarlow further argues that the disclosed method provides an improved replication of rowing because in actual rowing the rower is not assisted by the contraction of a spring or elastic cord during the "recovery" portion of the stroke. The rower must push the oar handle forward against wind and oarlock resistance in preparation for the next stroke. Tarlow asserts that the invention replicates that resistance.

A third non-elastic handle return strategy is disclosed in US patent, "Gravity Return Rowing Exercise Device" granted to Robert Edmondson. As stated in the patent document, the utilization of gravity (ie: a weight) to take up the chain and return the handle eliminates the inevitable variability of handle return force associated with an elastic cord system and thereby ensures consistency between machines.

Machines with a digital display calculate the user's power by measuring the speed of the flywheel during the stroke and then recording the rate at which it decelerates during the recovery. Using this and the known moment of inertia of the flywheel, the computer is able to calculate speed, power, distance and energy usage. Some ergometers can be connected to a personal computer using software, and data on individual exercise sessions can be collected and analysed. In addition, some software packages allows users to connect multiple ergometers either directly or over the internet for virtual races and workouts.

Motion Type

At the current state of the art, indoor rowers which utilize flywheel resistance can be categorized into two motion types. In both types, the rowing movement of the user causes the footrests and the seat to move further and closer apart in co-ordination with the user's stroke. The difference between the two types is in the movement, or absence of movement, of the footrests relative to ground.

The first type is characterized by the Dreissigacker/Williams device (referenced above). With this type the flywheel and footrests are fixed to a stationary frame, and the seat is free to slide fore and aft on a rail or rails integral to the stationary frame. Therefore, during use, the seat moves relative to the footrests and also relative to ground, while the flywheel and footrests remain stationary relative to ground. This type is sometimes referred to as a "stationary" or "fixed head" rowing ergometer.

The second type is characterized by the Rekers device. With this type, both the seat and the footrests are free to slide fore and aft on a rail or rails integral to a stationary frame. Therefore, during use, the seat and the footrests move relative to each other, and both also move relative to ground. This type is often referred to as a "dynamic" rowing ergometer, although "dynamically balanced" would be a more accurate description. The effect, for the user, is a more realistic "on the water" sensation than that provided by a "stationary" rowing ergometer because the "dynamically balanced" type more closely replicates actual rowing wherein the seat and the boat move relative to each other, and both move relative to the water.

Included within the "dynamically balanced" category are indoor rowers in which the footrests and flywheel are fixed to a moveable carriage, and also those in which the footrests alone are fixed to the moveable carriage, the carriage in both cases being free to slide fore and aft on a rail or rails integral to the stationary frame. The described device in which the flywheel is fixed to and moves with the carriage and footrests (the Rekers design) is sometimes referred to as a "floating head" rowing ergometer.

Indoor rowers which utilize a pivoting handle or handles to simulate a sweep or sculling stroke (thus referred to as "rowing simulators"), can be of the above described "stationary" or "dynamically balanced" type of rowing ergometer. The Coffey rowing machine, designed by Olympic silver medalist rower, Calvin Coffey, can be configured to enable a sweep or a sculling stroke, in either a "stationary" or "dynamically balanced" mode. The flywheel is positioned horizontally at the rear of the device, under the seat rails.

The Rekers rowing ergometer is described in the title of the patent document as "dynamically balanced", rather than simply "dynamic", as is common among users. "Dynamically balanced" is the accurate description, for the following reason: During the drive portion of the stroke, since the sliding carriage to which the footrests are attached, and the sliding seat, can both move independently fore and aft on a rail or rails, therefore the straightening of the user's legs causes the footrests to slide forward, and simultaneously causes the seat to slide rearward. However, since the combined mass of the seat and user is considerably greater than the combined mass of the footrests and sliding carriage (and flywheel, if it is part of the sliding footrests assembly), therefore the rearward movement of the seat and user, relative to ground, is much less than the forward movement of the footrests and carriage assembly, relative to ground. During the recovery portion of the stroke, this difference in mass has the same effect. The sliding footrests carriage, and the sliding seat carrying the user move proportionately the same distances relative to ground as during the drive as they return to their starting positions. Thus, during use, the combined mass of the footrest and sliding carriage, and the combined mass of the user and sliding seat, move towards and away from each other, as they oscillate about their common centre of gravity. To ensure the linked movement of these two masses remain centred on the device, the rail or rails upon which they slide are sloped upward slightly at their front and rear ends. Alternatively, elastic cords or springs attached to the seat and footrests can ensure such centering.

In addition to the aforementioned improved "on the water" sensation experienced by the user of a "dynamically balanced" rowing ergometer, there is a bio-mechanical advantage. Since, throughout all phases of the stroke, the user's mass moves only a small distance relative to ground, the user is not subject to the inertial stresses associated with the abrupt fore and aft directional changes experienced on a "stationary" rowing ergometer.

Damper Type

Piston resistance comes from hydraulic cylinders that are attached to the handles of the rowing machine. The length of the rower handles on this class of rower is typically adjustable, however, during the row the handle length is fixed which in turn fixes the trajectory that the hands must take on the stroke and return, thus making the stroke less accurate than is possible on the other types of resistance models where it is possible to emulate the difference in hand height on the stroke and return. Furthermore, many models in this class have a fixed seat position that eliminates the leg drive which is the foundation of competitive on water rowing technique. Because of the compact size of the pistons and mechanical simplicity of design, these models are typically not as large or as expensive as the others types.

Braked flywheel resistance models comprise magnetic, air and water resistance rowers. These machines are mechanically similar since all three types use a handle connected to a flywheel by rope, chain, or strap to provide resistance to the user – the types differ only in braking mechanism. Because the handle is attached to the resistance source by rope or similarly flexible media, the trajectory of the hands in the vertical plane is free making it possible for the rower to emulate the hand height difference between the stroke and the return. Most of these models have the characteristic sliding seat typical of competitive on-the-water boats.

> Magnetic resistance models control resistance by means of electromagnets that engage a mechanical brake with the flywheel. The magnetic braking system is quieter than the other braked flywheel types. The braking resistance is adjustable and energy can be accurately measured on this type of rower. The drawback of this type of resistance mechanism is that the resistance is constant; rowers using air or water resistance more accurately simulate actual rowing, where the resistance increases the harder the handle is pulled.
>
> Air resistance models use vanes on the flywheel to provide the flywheel braking needed to generate resistance. As the flywheel is spun faster, the air resistance increases. An adjustable vent can be used to control the volume of air moved by the vanes of the rotating flywheel, therefore a larger vent opening results in a higher resistance, and a smaller vent opening results in a lower resistance. The energy dissipated can be accurately calculated given the known moment of inertia of the flywheel and a tachometer to measure the deceleration of the flywheel. Air resistance rowing machines are most often used by sport rowers (particularly during the off season and inclement weather) and competitive indoor rowers. RowPerfect, Oartec, and Concept 2, are three manufacturers of this type of rowing machine.

Water resistance models consist of a paddle revolving in an enclosed tank of water. The mass and drag of the moving water creates the resistance. Proponents claim that this approach results in a more realistic action than possible with air or magnetic type machines. "Water-Rower" was the first company to manufacturer this type of rowing machine. The company was formed in the 1980's by John Duke, a US National Team rower, and inventor of the device (1989 US Patent US4884800A). At that time, in the patent record, there were a few prior art fluid resistance rowing machines, but they lacked the simplicity and elegance of the Duke design. From the 1989 patent Abstract: "rowing machine features a hollow container that holds a supply of water. Pulling on a drive cord during a pulling segment of a stroke rotates a paddle or like mechanism within the container to provide a momentum effect."

Rheological fluid resistance: In the patent record various exercise devices, including rowing machines, are depicted and described utilizing flywheels in which rotational resistance is controlled by varying the viscosity of a magnetically or electrically reactive fluid (magnetorheological or electrorheological fluid). It seems probable therefore that at some time commercially available rowing machines will include those with flywheels containing variable viscosity fluid.

Rowing machines with monitors calculate performance using an algorithm unique to the individual manufacturer; it will be affected by the type of resistance used and other factors.

Exercise

Indoor rowing primarily works the cardiovascular systems with typical workouts consisting of steady pieces of 20–40 minutes, although the standard trial distance for record attempts is 2000 m, which can take from five and a half minutes (best elite rowers) to nine minutes or more. Like other forms of cardio focused exercise, interval training is also commonly used in indoor rowing. While cardio-focused, rowing also stresses many muscle groups throughout the body anaerobically, thus rowing is often referred to as a strength-endurance sport.

Unlike high impact exercises, which can damage knees and the connective tissues of the lower body, rowing's most common injury site is the lower back. Proper technique is a necessity for staying injury free, with a focus on both mechanics and breathing, as correct rhythm, exhaling on the drive and inhaling on the recovery, is a stabilizing force for the upper body. Non-rowers commonly overemphasize the muscles of the upper body, while correct technique uses the large muscle of the thighs to drive much of the stroke. Also, good technique requires that the angle of the upper body is never too far forward, nor too far back, both of which jeopardize the lower back and compression injuries on the knees and hip flexor muscles. Proper technique however, can only be achieved if the design of the exercise equipment enables proper technique. The ubiquitous rigid, single-piece handle does not follow the natural movement of a user's hands, wrists, and forearms as the stroke progresses. It does not ensure or enable the bio-mechanically correct alignment of the hands, wrists, and forearms with the direction of the applied force. Typically, the user finishes the stroke with the wrists in an angulated position. It is incorrect to criticize this as "bad technique", when the equipment itself is the cause. Through no fault of their own, regular users of indoor rowers equipped with the standard single-piece handle, are prone to repetitive strain injury and chronic wrist pain.

In addition to the high levels of fitness attained, rowing is an intense calorie-burning exercise. The late Dr. Fritz Hagerman, Professor of biomedical science and a leading researcher in rowing physiology, determined that "you burn more calories in rowing than any other activity. Cross-country skiing comes closest. At standard submaximal levels of exercise, rowing will burn calories at a rate 10-12% higher than running, and 15-20% higher than cycling." Although rowers with less ability and training will burn fewer calories, the ergometer is an excellent tool for use in a weight-loss program.

The standard measurement of speed on an ergometer is generally known as the "split", or the amount of time in minutes and seconds required to travel 500 metres (1,600 ft) at the current pace — a split of 2:00 represents a speed of two minutes per 500 metres, or about 4.17 m/s (15.0 km/h). The split does not necessarily correspond to how many strokes the rower takes (the "rating") since strokes can vary in power.

Ergometer Testing

Ergometer tests are used by rowing coaches to evaluate rowers and is part of athlete selection for many senior and junior national rowing teams. During a test, rowers will row a set distance and try to clock the fastest time possible, or a set time and try to row the longest distance possible. The most common distances for erg tests are 1000, 2000, 5000, 6000 or 10000 metres. The most common times for erg tests are 3 min, 5 min, 20 min, 30 min, and 1 hour.

Rowing Technique

Rowing technique on the erg broadly follows the same pattern as that of a normal rowing stroke on water, but with minor modifications: it is not necessary to "tap down" at the finish, since there are no blades to extract from water; but many who also row on water do this anyway. Also, the rigid, single-piece handle enables neither a sweep nor a sculling stroke. The oar handle during a sweep stroke follows a long arc, while the oar handles during a sculling stroke follow two arcs. The standard handle does neither. But regardless of this, to reduce the chance of injury, an exercise machine should enable a bio-mechanically correct movement of the user. The handle is the interface between the human and the machine, and should adapt to the natural movement of the user, not the user to the machine, as is now the case. During competitions an exaggerated finish is often used, whereby the hands are pulled further up the chest than would be possible on the water, resulting in a steep angulation of the wrists - but even with a normal stroke, stop-action images show wrist angulation at the finish, evidence that the standard rigid, single-piece handle does not allow the user to maintain a bio-mechanically correct alignment of hands, wrists, and forearms in the direction of applied force. On the Concept 2 website "Forum", many regular users of the indoor rower have complained of chronic wrist pain. Some have rigged handgrips with flexible straps to enable their hands, wrists, and forearms to maintain proper alignment, and thereby reduce the possibility of repetitive strain injury. Rowing machine manufacturers have ignored this problem.

Rowing on an ergometer requires four basics phases to complete one stroke; the catch, the drive, the finish and the recovery. The catch is the initial part of the stroke. The drive is where the power from the rower is generated while the finish is the final part of the stroke. Then, the recovery is the initial phase to begin taking a new stroke. The phases repeat until a time duration or a distance is completed.

Catch

Knees are bent with the shins in a vertical position. The back should be roughly parallel to the thigh without hyperflexion (leaning forward too far). The arms and shoulders should be extended forward and relaxed. The arms should be level.

Drive

The drive is initiated by the extension of the legs; the body remains in the catch posture at this point of the drive. As the legs continue to full extension, the rower engages the core to begin the motion of the body levering backward, adding to the work of the legs. When the legs are flat, the rower begins to pull the handle toward the chest with their arms while keeping their arms straight and parallel to the floor.

Finish

The legs are at full extension and flat. The shoulders are slightly behind the pelvis, and the arms are in full contraction with the elbows bent and hands against the chest below the nipples. The back of the rower is still maintained in an upright posture and wrists should be flat.

Recovery

The recovery is a slow slide back to the initial part of the stroke, it gives the rower time to recover from the previous stroke. During the recovery the actions are in reverse order of the drive. The arms are fully extended so that they are straight. The torso is engaged to move forward back over the pelvis. Weight transfers from the back of the seat to the front of the seat at this time. When the hands come over the knees, the legs contract back towards the foot stretcher. Slowly the back becomes more parallel to the thighs until the recovery becomes the catch.

High Knees

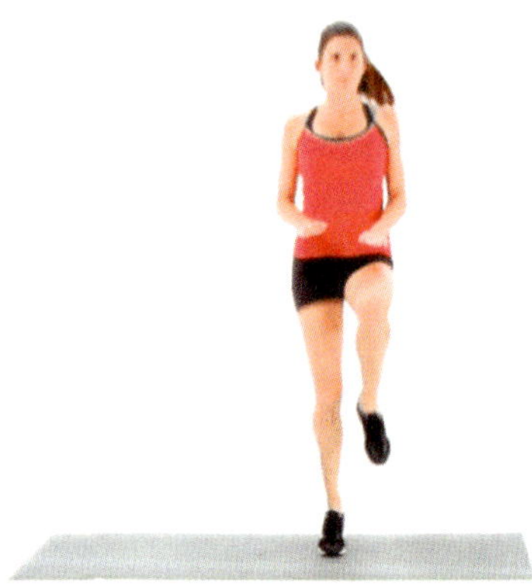

High knees combine the typical running motion with exaggerated knee lifts. They are often used by runners and other athletes to improve running form as well as lower body speed, power, and flexibility. Perform high knees as a component of your warm-up or prolong the exercise and add them to your workout routine to really get your heart rate going. There are several variations of the high knees exercise you can implement into your fitness routine.

Basic High Knees

Basic high knees can be performed while running in place or moving over a distance. Stand in place with your feet hip-width apart. Drive your right knee toward your chest and quickly place it back on the ground. Follow immediately by driving your left knee toward your chest. Continue to alternate knees as quickly as you can. If you are incorporating this exercise into your warm-up, begin with slower, controlled movements to prevent a pulling a muscle. Perform this exercise for a designated amount of time or over a specified distance. For example, you could run in place with high knees for one minute or run 30 feet with high knees.

High Knees is an awesome cardio exercise that works your legs and core while giving you a great cardiovascular move that gets your heart rate up anytime, anywhere. If you've already been incorporating high knees into your workout routine, then consider switching them up with other high knee equivalents that can target similar muscles, such as Steam Engine, High Knee March, Butt Kicks, and Power Skips!

Steam Engine

The steam engine is a simple exercise that combines high knees with arm and upper-body movement. This exercise is great for building strength and endurance in your hip flexors and abdominal muscles. Stand with your feet hip width apart, interlock your fingers behind your head and open your elbows to the side. In a controlled manner, drive your right knee up to the front. At the same time, twist your torso and touch your left elbow to the raised knee. Pause at the top of the movement and then return your right foot to the floor. Repeat the lift with your left leg, touching your right elbow to your left knee. Continue to alternate knees until your muscles fatigue.

High Knee March

The high knee march is similar to the steam engine exercise but is a more dynamic movement. Stand with your feet slightly apart, your weight concentrated in the balls of your feet and your arms relaxed at your sides. Lift your left knee high while bringing your heel toward your glutes and keeping your toes up. Drive your leg back toward the ground, taking a small step forward. Repeat the movement with your right leg. Continue to march until you have covered a desired specified distance.

Skipping

Skipping is not just for kids, but also for athletes looking to improve power and upward acceleration. This exercise is a variation of the basic high knees exercise but requires much more explosiveness. Stand with your feet hip width apart and bend your elbows to 90 degrees with your arms at your sides. Drive your right knee and left arm up while exploding upward off your left leg. Land on your left leg and then immediately drive your left knee and right arm up while pushing off of your right foot. With each skip, propel yourself upward as high as possible while driving the lifted knee toward your chest. Continue to skip in this manner until you have covered a desired specified distance.

Calorie Burnt During High Knees

People often ask how many calories they are burning in their workouts, and while we wish it was as simple as saying certain exercises burn a specific amount of calories, it generally boils down to how hard you're working. High Knees will generally burn about 100 calories for every 10 minutes you are working at a moderate to intense fitness level. Just keep your intensity up and make sure you are breathing through your mouth. Bottom line—the harder you work, the more calories you burn.

Benefits

- Develops strength and endurance of the hip flexors, the muscles that lift the knees and prevent plodding in the running stride
- Develops strength and endurance of the quads
- Stretches the hip extensors, which include the gluteal muscles
- These benefits lead to a longer stride for faster, more efficient running.

Outdoor Aerobic Exercises

Boxing

Boxing is a combat game played throughout the world. The history of the combat sports game seems to be more interesting and the participation of people get increased day by day. It is a pre-historic game which founds its origin in ancient Greek period. Generally, boxing is played by two numbers of players where people fight, knocks each other on proper techniques.

The origin of boxing game was found to be in the ancient Greek period and then later by ancient Romans. It was found that during that period they had sports called pugilism which is also referred as boxing. This type of sports event was said to be more popular and most of the people shows their interest in developing the skill and knowledge in the field. Energetic, professional trainers were exercised to provide training and due to the interest of people, it was widely spread throughout the world. People who engaged in the sports play through by fighting each other with their fists and hands. Adequate training is required to the participants to play the successfully and technically.

To play the event, the boxer requires boxing equipments to protect him against damages and injuries. Different sorts of combat equipments are available and the customer should have to make use of it as per his requirement. Some of the equipments the players popularly used are gloves, headgear, shoes, punching bags, rings, mouthpiece, handwraps and even more. These gears will be highly helpful to the players because these instruments will protect them against damages at the time of fighting against one another. Large numbers of players shows their interest and learns the programs enthusiastically.

Rules

The *Marquess of Queensberry rules* have been the general rules governing modern boxing.

A boxing match typically consists of a determined number of three-minute rounds, a total of up to 9 to 12 rounds. A minute is typically spent between each round with the fighters in their assigned corners receiving advice and attention from their coach and staff. The fight is controlled by a referee who works within the ring to judge and control the conduct of the fighters, rule on their ability to fight safely, count knocked-down fighters, and rule on fouls.

Up to three judges are typically present at ringside to score the bout and assign points to the boxers, based on punches and elbows that connect, defense, knockdowns, hugging and other, more subjective, measures. Because of the open-ended style of boxing judging, many fights have controversial results, in which one or both fighters believe they have been "robbed" or unfairly denied a victory. Each fighter has an assigned corner of the ring, where his or her coach, as well as one or more "seconds" may administer to the fighter at the beginning of the fight and between rounds. Each boxer enters into the ring from their assigned corners at the beginning of each round and must cease fighting and return to their corner at the signalled end of each round.

A bout in which the predetermined number of rounds passes is decided by the judges, and is said to "go the distance". The fighter with the higher score at the end of the fight is ruled the winner. With three judges, unanimous and split decisions are possible, as are draws. A boxer may win the bout before a decision is reached through a knock-out; such bouts are said to have ended "inside the distance". If a fighter is knocked down during the fight, determined by whether the boxer touches the canvas floor of the ring with any part of their body other than the feet as a result of the opponent's punch and not a slip, as determined by the referee, the referee begins counting until the fighter returns to his or her feet and can continue. Some jurisdictions require the referee to count to eight regardless of if the fighter gets up before.

Should the referee count to ten, then the knocked-down boxer is ruled "knocked out" (whether unconscious or not) and the other boxer is ruled the winner by knockout (KO). A "technical knockout" (TKO) is possible as well, and is ruled by the referee, fight doctor, or a fighter's corner if a fighter is unable to safely continue to fight, based upon injuries or being judged unable to effectively defend themselves. Many jurisdictions and sanctioning agencies also have a "three-knockdown rule", in which three knockdowns in a given round result in a TKO. A TKO is considered a knockout in a fighter's record. A "standing eight" count rule may also be in effect. This gives the referee the right to step in and administer a count of eight to a fighter that he or she feels may be in danger, even if no knockdown has taken place. After counting the referee will observe the fighter, and decide if he or she is fit to continue. For scoring purposes, a standing eight count is treated as a knockdown.

In general, boxers are prohibited from hitting below the belt, holding, tripping, pushing, biting, or spitting. The boxer's shorts are raised so the opponent is not allowed to hit to the groin area with intent to cause pain or injury. Failure to abide by the former may result in a foul. They also are prohibited from kicking, head-butting, or hitting with any part of the arm other than the knuckles of a closed fist (including hitting with the elbow, shoulder or forearm, as well as with open gloves, the wrist, the inside, back or side of the hand). They are prohibited as well from hitting the back, back of the head or neck (called a "rabbit-punch") or the kidneys. They are prohibited from holding the ropes for support when punching, holding an opponent while punching, or ducking below the belt of their opponent (dropping below the waist of your opponent, no matter the distance between).

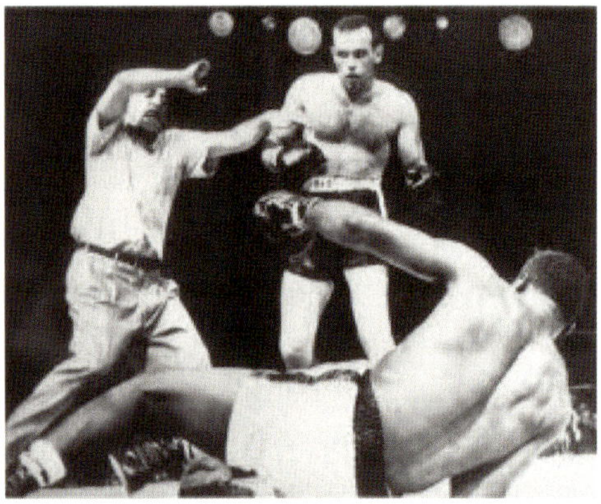

Ingemar Johansson of Sweden KO's heavyweight champion Floyd Patterson.

If a "clinch" – a defensive move in which a boxer wraps his or her opponents arms and holds on to create a pause – is broken by the referee, each fighter must take a full step back before punching again (alternatively, the referee may direct the fighters to "punch out" of the clinch). When a boxer is knocked down, the other boxer must immediately cease fighting and move to the furthest neutral corner of the ring until the referee has either ruled a knockout or called for the fight to continue.

Violations of these rules may be ruled "fouls" by the referee, who may issue warnings, deduct points, or disqualify an offending boxer, causing an automatic loss, depending on the seriousness and intentionality of the foul. An intentional foul that causes injury that prevents a fight from continuing usually causes the boxer who committed it to be disqualified. A fighter who suffers an accidental low-blow may be given up to five minutes to recover, after which they may be ruled knocked out if they are unable to continue. Accidental fouls that cause injury ending a bout may lead to a "no contest" result, or else cause the fight to go to a decision if enough rounds (typically four or more, or at least three in a four-round fight) have passed.

Unheard of in the modern era, but common during the early 20th Century in North America, a "newspaper decision (NWS)" might be made after a no decision bout had ended. A "no decision" bout occurred when, by law or by pre-arrangement of the fighters, if both boxers were still standing at the fight's conclusion and there was no knockout, no official decision was rendered and neither boxer was declared the winner. But this did not prevent the pool of ringside newspaper reporters from declaring a consensus result among themselves and printing a newspaper decision in their publications. Officially, however, a "no decision" bout resulted in neither boxer winning or losing. Boxing historians sometimes use these unofficial newspaper decisions in compiling fight records for illustrative purposes only. Often, media outlets covering a match will personally score the match, and post their scores as an independent sentence in their report.

Professional vs. Amateur Boxing

Throughout the 17th to 19th centuries, boxing bouts were motivated by money, as the fighters competed for prize money, promoters controlled the gate, and spectators bet on the result. The modern Olympic movement revived interest in amateur sports, and amateur boxing became an Olympic sport in 1908. In their current form, Olympic and other amateur bouts are typically limited to three or four rounds, scoring is computed by points based on the number of clean blows landed, regardless of impact, and fighters wear protective headgear, reducing the number of injuries, knockdowns, and knockouts. Currently scoring blows in amateur boxing are subjectively counted by ringside judges, but the Australian Institute for Sport has demonstrated a prototype of an Automated Boxing Scoring System, which introduces scoring objectivity, improves safety, and arguably makes the sport more interesting to spectators. Professional boxing remains by far the most popular form of the sport globally, though amateur boxing is dominant in Cuba and some former Soviet republics. For most fighters, an amateur career, especially at the Olympics, serves to develop skills and gain experience in preparation for a professional career. Western boxers typically participate in one Olympics and then turn pro, Cubans and other socialist countries have an opportunity to collect multiple medals. In 2016, professional boxers were admitted in the Olympic Games and other tournaments sanctioned by AIBA. This was done in part to level the playing field and give all of the athletes the same opportunities government-sponsored boxers from socialist countries and post-Soviet republics have. However, professional organizations strongly opposed that decision.

Amateur Boxing

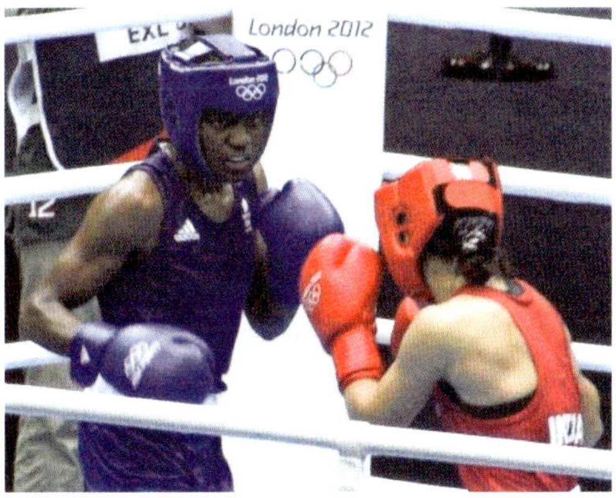

Nicola Adams is the first female boxer to win an Olympic gold medal.

Amateur boxing may be found at the collegiate level, at the Olympic Games and Commonwealth Games, and in many other venues sanctioned by amateur boxing associations. Amateur boxing has a point scoring system that measures the number of clean blows landed rather than physical damage. Bouts consist of three rounds of three minutes in the Olympic and Commonwealth Games, and three rounds of three minutes in a national ABA (Amateur Boxing Association) bout, each with a one-minute interval between rounds.

Competitors wear protective headgear and gloves with a white strip or circle across the knuckle. There are cases however, where white ended gloves are not required but any solid color may be worn. The white end just is a way to make it easier for judges to score clean hits. Each competitor must have their hands properly wrapped, pre-fight, for added protection on their hands and for added cushion under the gloves. Gloves worn by the fighters must be twelve ounces in weight unless the fighters weigh under 165 pounds (75 kg), thus allowing them to wear ten ounce gloves. A punch is considered a scoring punch only when the boxers connect with the white portion of the gloves. Each punch that lands cleanly on the head or torso with sufficient force is awarded a point. A referee monitors the fight to ensure that competitors use only legal blows. A belt worn over the torso represents the lower limit of punches – any boxer repeatedly landing low blows below the belt is disqualified. Referees also ensure that the boxers don't use holding tactics to prevent the opponent from swinging. If this occurs, the referee separates the opponents and orders them to continue boxing. Repeated holding can result in a boxer being penalized or ultimately disqualified. Referees will stop the bout if a boxer is seriously injured, if one boxer is significantly dominating the other or if the score is severely imbalanced. Amateur bouts which end this way may be noted as "RSC" (referee stopped contest) with notations for an outclassed opponent (RSCO), outscored opponent (RSCOS), injury (RSCI) or head injury (RSCH).

Professional Boxing

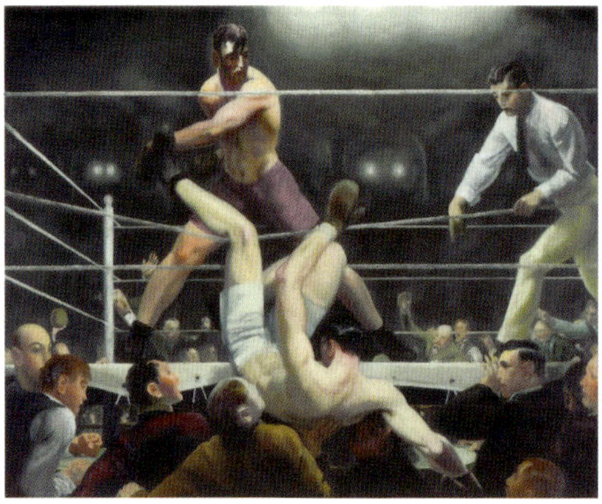

Firpo sending Dempsey outside the ring.

Professional bouts are usually much longer than amateur bouts, typically ranging from ten to twelve rounds, though four-round fights are common for less experienced fighters or club fighters. There are also some two- and three-round professional bouts, especially in Australia. Through the early 20th century, it was common for fights to have unlimited rounds, ending only when one fighter quit, benefiting high-energy fighters like Jack Dempsey. Fifteen rounds remained the internationally recognized limit for championship fights for most of the 20th century until the early 1980s, when the death of boxer Kim Duk-koo eventually prompted the World Boxing Council and other organizations sanctioning professional boxing to reduce the limit to twelve rounds.

Headgear is not permitted in professional bouts, and boxers are generally allowed to take much more damage before a fight is halted. At any time, the referee may stop the contest if he believes that one participant cannot defend himself due to injury. In that case, the other participant is awarded a technical knockout win. A technical knockout would also be awarded if a fighter lands a punch that opens a cut on the opponent, and the opponent is later deemed not fit to continue by a doctor because of the cut. For this reason, fighters often employ cutmen, whose job is to treat cuts between rounds so that the boxer is able to continue despite the cut. If a boxer simply quits fighting, or if his corner stops the fight, then the winning boxer is also awarded a technical knockout victory. In contrast with amateur boxing, professional male boxers have to be bare-chested.

Boxing Styles

Definition of style

"Style" is often defined as the strategic approach a fighter takes during a bout. No two fighters' styles are alike, as each is determined by that individual's physical and mental attributes. Three main styles exist in boxing: outside fighter ("boxer"), brawler (or "slugger"), and Inside fighter ("swarmer"). These styles may be divided into several special subgroups, such as counter puncher, etc. The main philosophy of the styles is, that each style has an advantage over one, but disadvantage over the other one. It follows the rock-paper-scissors scenario - boxer beats brawler, brawler beats swarmer, and swarmer beats boxer.

Boxer/Out-fighter

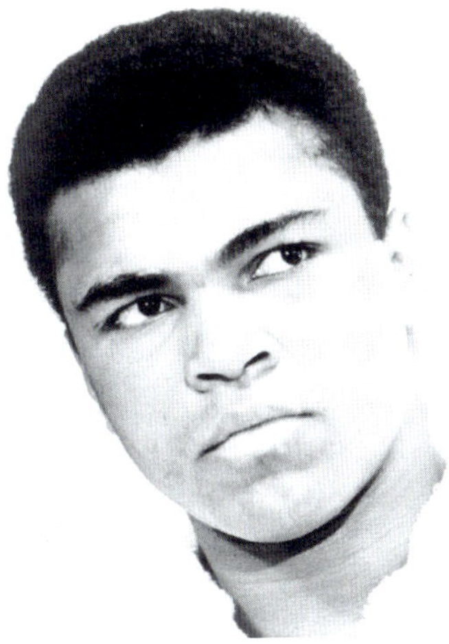

Heavyweight champion Muhammad Ali was a typical example of an out-fighter.

A classic "boxer" or stylist (also known as an "out-fighter") seeks to maintain distance between himself and his opponent, fighting with faster, longer range punches, most notably the jab, and gradually wearing his opponent down. Due to this reliance on weaker punches, out-fighters tend to win by point decisions rather than by knockout, though some out-fighters have notable knockout records. They are often regarded as the best boxing strategists due to their ability to control the pace of the fight and lead their opponent, methodically wearing him down and exhibiting more skill and finesse than a brawler. Out-fighters need reach, hand speed, reflexes, and footwork.

Notable out-fighters include Muhammad Ali, Larry Holmes, Joe Calzaghe, Wilfredo Gómez, Salvador Sanchez, Cecilia Brækhus, Gene Tunney, Ezzard Charles, Willie Pep, Meldrick Taylor, Ricardo Lopez, Floyd Mayweather Jr., Roy Jones Jr., Sugar Ray Leonard, Miguel Vazquez, Sergio "Maravilla" Martínez, Vitali Klitschko, Wladimir Klitschko and Guillermo Rigondeaux. This style was also used by fictional boxer Apollo Creed.

Boxer-puncher

A boxer-puncher is a well-rounded boxer who is able to fight at close range with a combination of technique and power, often with the ability to knock opponents out with a combination and in some instances a single shot. Their movement and tactics are similar to that of an out-fighter (although they are generally not as mobile as an out-fighter), but instead of winning by decision, they tend to wear their opponents down using combinations and then move in to score the knockout. A boxer must be well rounded to be effective using this style.

Notable boxer-punchers include Muhammad Ali, Canelo Álvarez, Wladimir Klitschko, Vasyl Lomachenko, Lennox Lewis, Joe Louis, Wilfredo Gómez, Oscar de la Hoya, Archie Moore, Miguel Cotto, Nonito Donaire, Sam Langford, Henry Armstrong, Sugar Ray Robinson, Tony Zale, Carlos Monzón, Alexis Argüello, Erik Morales, Terry Norris, Marco Antonio Barrera, Naseem Hamed and Thomas Hearns.

Counter Puncher

Counter punchers are slippery, defensive style fighters who often rely on their opponent's mistakes in order to gain the advantage, whether it be on the score cards or more preferably a knockout. They use their well-rounded defense to avoid or block shots and then immediately catch the opponent off guard with a well placed and timed punch. A fight with a skilled counter-puncher can turn into a war of attrition, where each shot landed is a battle in itself. Thus, fighting against counter punchers requires constant feinting and the ability to avoid telegraphing one's attacks. To be truly successful using this style they must have good reflexes, a high level of prediction and awareness, pinpoint accuracy and speed, both in striking and in footwork.

Notable counter punchers include Muhammad Ali, Joe Calzaghe, Vitali Klitschko, Evander Holyfield, Max Schmeling, Chris Byrd, Jim Corbett, Jack Johnson, Bernard Hopkins, Laszlo Papp, Jerry Quarry, Anselmo Moreno, James Toney, Marvin Hagler, Juan Manuel Márquez, Humberto Soto, Floyd Mayweather Jr., Roger Mayweather, Pernell Whitaker, Sergio Gabriel Martinez and Guillermo Rigondeaux. This style of boxing is also used by fictional boxer Little Mac.

Counter punchers usually wear their opponents down by causing them to miss their punches. The more the opponent misses, the faster they tire, and the psychological effects of being unable to land a hit will start to sink in. The counter puncher often tries to outplay their opponent entirely, not just in a physical sense, but also in a mental and emotional sense. This style can be incredibly difficult, especially against seasoned fighters, but winning a fight without getting hit is often worth the pay-off. They usually try to stay away from the center of the ring, in order to outmaneuver and chip away at their opponents. A large advantage in counter-hitting is the forward momentum of the attacker, which drives them further into your return strike. As such, knockouts are more common than one would expect from a defensive style.

Brawler/Slugger

A brawler is a fighter who generally lacks finesse and footwork in the ring, but makes up for it through sheer punching power. Many brawlers tend to lack mobility, preferring a less mobile, more stable platform and have difficulty pursuing fighters who are fast on their feet. They may also have a tendency to ignore combination punching in favor of continuous beat-downs with one hand and by throwing slower, more powerful single punches (such as hooks and uppercuts). Their slowness and predictable punching pattern (single punches with obvious leads) often leaves them open to counter punches, so successful brawlers must be able to absorb substantial amounts of punishment. However, not all brawler/slugger fighters are not mobile; some can move around and switch styles if needed but still have the brawler/slugger style such as Wilfredo Gómez, Prince Naseem Hamed and Danny García.

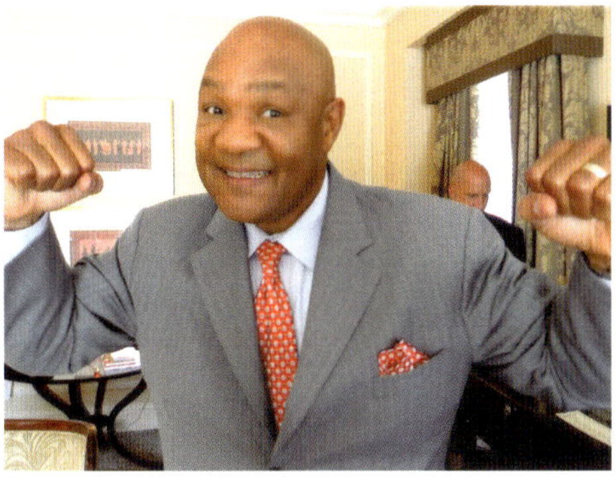

Famous brawler George Foreman

A brawler's most important assets are power and chin (the ability to absorb punishment while remaining able to continue boxing). Examples of this style include George Foreman, Rocky Marciano, Julio César Chávez, Roberto Duran, Danny García, Wilfredo Gómez, Sonny Liston, John L. Sullivan, Max Baer, Prince Naseem Hamed, Ray Mancini, David Tua, Arturo Gatti, Micky Ward, Brandon Ríos, Ruslan Provodnikov, Michael Katsidis, James Kirkland, Marcos Maidana, Jake LaMotta, Manny Pacquiao, and Ireland's John Duddy. This style of boxing was also used by fictional boxers Rocky Balboa and James "Clubber" Lang.

Brawlers tend to be more predictable and easy to hit but usually fare well enough against other fighting styles because they train to take punches very well. They often have a higher chance than other fighting styles to score a knockout against their opponents because they focus on landing big, powerful hits, instead of smaller, faster attacks. Oftentimes they place focus on training on their upper body instead of their entire body, to increase power and endurance. They also aim to intimidate their opponents because of their power, stature and ability to take a punch.

Swarmer/In-fighter

In-fighters/swarmers (sometimes called "pressure fighters") attempt to stay close to an opponent, throwing intense flurries and combinations of hooks and uppercuts. Mainly Mexican, Irish, Irish-American, Puerto Rican, and Mexican-American boxers popularized this style. A successful in-fighter often needs a good "chin" because swarming usually involves being hit with many jabs before they can maneuver inside where they are more effective. In-fighters operate best at close range because they are generally shorter and have less reach than their opponents and thus are more effective at a short distance where the longer arms of their opponents make punching awkward. However, several fighters tall for their division have been relatively adept at in-fighting as well as out-fighting.

The essence of a swarmer is non-stop aggression. Many short in-fighters utilize their stature to their advantage, employing a bob-and-weave defense by bending at the waist to slip underneath or to the sides of incoming punches. Unlike blocking, causing an opponent to miss a punch disrupts his balance, this permits forward movement past the opponent's extended arm and keeps the hands free to counter. A distinct advantage that in-fighters have is when throwing uppercuts, they can channel their entire bodyweight behind the punch; Mike Tyson was famous for throwing devastating uppercuts. Marvin Hagler was known for his hard "chin", punching power, body attack and the stalking of his opponents. Some in-fighters, like Mike Tyson, have been known for being notoriously hard to hit. The key to a swarmer is aggression, endurance, chin, and bobbing-and-weaving.

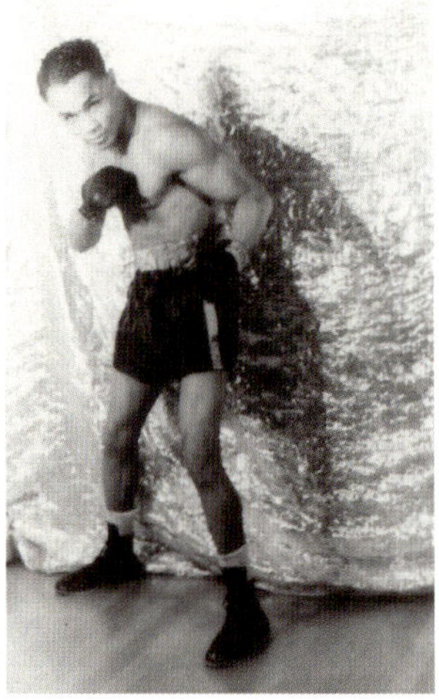

Henry Armstrong was known for his aggressive, non-stop assault style of fighting.

Notable in-fighters include Henry Armstrong, Aaron Pryor, Julio César Chávez, Jack Dempsey, Shawn Porter, Miguel Cotto, Joe Frazier, Danny García, Mike Tyson, Manny Pacquiao, Rocky Marciano, Wayne McCullough, Gerry Penalosa, Harry Greb, David Tua, Ricky Hatton and Gennady Golovkin. This style was also used by the Street Fighter character Balrog.

Combinations of Styles

All fighters have primary skills with which they feel most comfortable, but truly elite fighters are often able to incorporate auxiliary styles when presented with a particular challenge. For example, an out-fighter will sometimes plant his feet and counter punch, or a slugger may have the stamina to pressure fight with his power punches.

Style Matchups

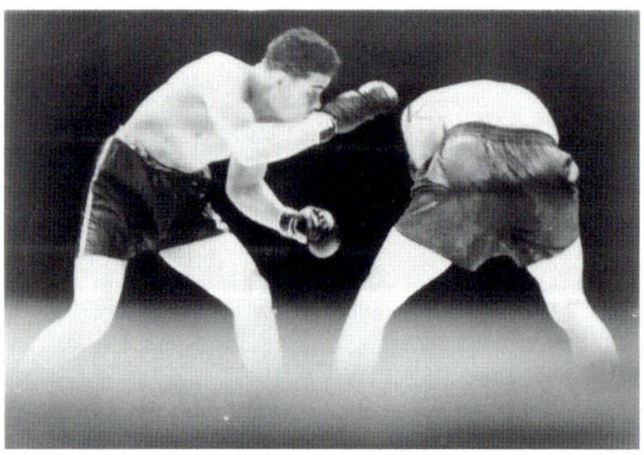

There is a generally accepted rule of thumb about the success each of these boxing styles has against the others. In general, an in-fighter has an advantage over an out-fighter, an out-fighter has an advantage over a brawler, and a brawler has an advantage over an in-fighter; these form a cycle with each style being stronger relative to one, and weaker relative to another, with none dominating, as in rock-paper-scissors. Naturally, many other factors, such as the skill level and training of the combatants, determine the outcome of a fight, but the widely held belief in this relationship among the styles is embodied in the cliché amongst boxing fans and writers that "styles make fights."

Brawlers tend to overcome swarmers or in-fighters because, in trying to get close to the slugger, the in-fighter will invariably have to walk straight into the guns of the much harder-hitting brawler, so, unless the former has a very good chin and the latter's stamina is poor, the brawler's superior power will carry the day. A famous example of this type of match-up advantage would be George Foreman's knockout victory over Joe Frazier in their original bout "The Sunshine Showdown".

Although in-fighters struggle against heavy sluggers, they typically enjoy more success against out-fighters or boxers. Out-fighters prefer a slower fight, with some distance between themselves and the opponent. The in-fighter tries to close that gap and unleash furious flurries. On the inside, the out-fighter loses a lot of his combat effectiveness, because he cannot throw the hard punches. The in-fighter is generally successful in this case, due to his intensity in advancing on his opponent and his good agility, which makes him difficult to evade. For example, the swarming Joe Frazier, though easily dominated by the slugger George Foreman, was able to create many more problems for the boxer Muhammad Ali in their three fights. Joe Louis, after retirement, admitted that he hated being crowded, and that swarmers like untied/undefeated champ Rocky Marciano would have caused him style problems even in his prime.

The boxer or out-fighter tends to be most successful against a brawler, whose slow speed (both hand and foot) and poor technique makes him an easy target to hit for the faster out-fighter. The out-fighter's main concern is to stay alert, as the brawler only needs to land one good punch to finish the fight. If the out-fighter can avoid those power punches, he can often wear the brawler down with fast jabs, tiring him out. If he is successful enough, he may even apply extra pressure in the later rounds in an attempt to achieve a knockout. Most classic boxers, such as Muhammad Ali, enjoyed their best successes against sluggers.

An example of a style matchup was the historical fight of Julio César Chávez, a swarmer or in-fighter, against Meldrick Taylor, the boxer or out-fighter. The match was nicknamed "Thunder Meets Lightning" as an allusion to punching power of Chávez and blinding speed of Taylor. Chávez was the epitome of the "Mexican" style of boxing. Taylor's hand and foot speed and boxing abilities gave him the early advantage, allowing him to begin building a large lead on points. Chávez remained relentless in his pursuit of Taylor and due to his greater punching power Chávez slowly punished Taylor. Coming into the later rounds, Taylor was bleeding from the mouth, his entire face was swollen, the bones around his eye socket had been broken, he had swallowed a considerable amount of his own blood, and as he grew tired, Taylor was increasingly forced into exchanging blows with Chávez, which only gave Chávez a greater chance to cause damage. While there was little doubt that Taylor had solidly won the first three quarters of the fight, the question at hand was whether he would survive the final quarter. Going into the final round, Taylor held a secure lead on the scorecards of two of the three judges. Chávez would have to knock Taylor out to claim a victory, whereas Taylor merely needed to stay away from the Mexican legend. However, Taylor did not stay away, but continued to trade blows with Chávez. As he did so, Taylor showed signs of extreme exhaustion, and every tick of the clock brought Taylor closer to victory unless Chávez could knock him out. With about a minute left in the round, Chávez hit Taylor squarely with several hard punches and stayed on the attack, continuing to hit Taylor with well-placed shots. Finally, with about 25 seconds to go, Chávez landed a hard right hand that caused Taylor to stagger forward towards a corner, forcing Chávez back ahead of him.

Suddenly Chávez stepped around Taylor, positioning him so that Taylor was trapped in the corner, with no way to escape from Chávez' desperate final flurry. Chávez then nailed Taylor with a tremendous right hand that dropped the younger man. By using the ring ropes to pull himself up, Taylor managed to return to his feet and was given the mandatory 8-count. Referee Richard Steele asked Taylor twice if he was able to continue fighting, but Taylor failed to answer. Steele then concluded that Taylor was unfit to continue and signaled that he was ending the fight, resulting in a TKO victory for Chávez with only two seconds to go in the bout.

Equipment

Since boxing involves forceful, repetitive punching, precautions must be taken to prevent damage to bones in the hand. Most trainers do not allow boxers to train and spar without wrist wraps and boxing gloves. Hand wraps are used to secure the bones in the hand, and the gloves are used to protect the hands from blunt injury, allowing boxers to throw punches with more force than if they did not utilise them. Gloves have been required in competition since the late nineteenth century, though modern boxing gloves are much heavier than those worn by early twentieth-century fighters. Prior to a bout, both boxers agree upon the weight of gloves to be used in the bout, with the understanding that lighter gloves allow heavy punchers to inflict more damage. The brand of gloves can also affect the impact of punches, so this too is usually stipulated before a bout. Both sides are allowed to inspect the wraps and gloves of the opponent to help ensure both are within agreed upon specifications and no tampering has taken place.

A mouthguard is important to protect the teeth and gums from injury, and to cushion the jaw, resulting in a decreased chance of knockout. Both fighters must wear soft soled shoes to reduce the damage from accidental (or intentional) stepping on feet. While older boxing boots more commonly resembled those of a professional wrestler, modern boxing shoes and boots tend to be quite similar to their amateur wrestling counterparts.

Boxers practice their skills on two basic types of punching bags. A small, tear-drop-shaped "speed bag" is used to hone reflexes and repetitive punching skills, while a large cylindrical "heavy bag" filled with sand, a synthetic substitute, or water is used to practice power punching and body blows. In addition to these distinctive pieces of equipment, boxers also utilize sport-nonspecific training equipment to build strength, speed, agility, and stamina. Common training equipment includes free weights, rowing machines, jump rope, and medicine balls.

Boxing matches typically take place in a boxing ring, a raised platform surrounded by ropes attached to posts rising in each corner. The term "ring" has come to be used as a metaphor for many aspects of prize fighting in general.

Technique

Stance

The modern boxing stance differs substantially from the typical boxing stances of the 19th and early 20th centuries. The modern stance has a more upright vertical-armed guard, as opposed to the more horizontal, knuckles-facing-forward guard adopted by early 20th century hook users such as Jack Johnson.

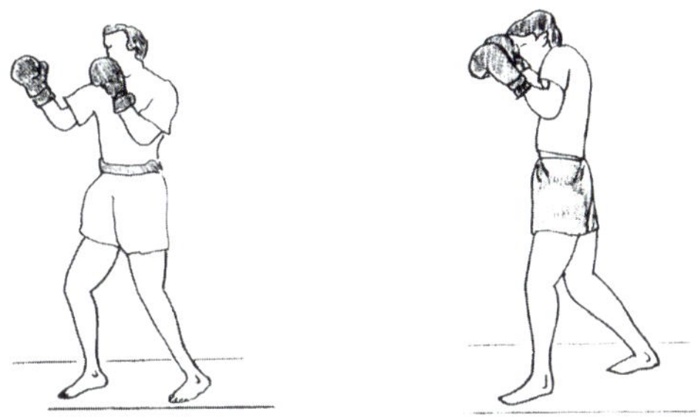

Upright stance Semi-crouch Full crouch

In a fully upright stance, the boxer stands with the legs shoulder-width apart and the rear foot a half-step in front of the lead man. Right-handed or orthodox boxers lead with the left foot and fist (for most penetration power). Both feet are parallel, and the right heel is off the ground. The lead (left) fist is held vertically about six inches in front of the face at eye level. The rear (right) fist is held beside the chin and the elbow tucked against the ribcage to protect the body. The chin is tucked into the chest to avoid punches to the jaw which commonly cause knock-outs and is often kept slightly off-center. Wrists are slightly bent to avoid damage when punching and the elbows are kept tucked in to protect the ribcage. Some boxers fight from a crouch, leaning forward and keeping their feet closer together. The stance described is considered the "textbook" stance and fighters are encouraged to change it around once it's been mastered as a base. Case in point, many fast fighters have their hands down and have almost exaggerated footwork, while brawlers or bully fighters tend to slowly stalk their opponents.

Left-handed or southpaw fighters use a mirror image of the orthodox stance, which can create problems for orthodox fighters unaccustomed to receiving jabs, hooks, or crosses from the opposite side. The southpaw stance, conversely, is vulnerable to a straight right hand.

North American fighters tend to favor a more balanced stance, facing the opponent almost squarely, while many European fighters stand with their torso turned more to the side. The positioning of the hands may also vary, as some fighters prefer to have both hands raised in front of the face, risking exposure to body shots.

Modern boxers can sometimes be seen tapping their cheeks or foreheads with their fists in order to remind themselves to keep their hands up (which becomes difficult during long bouts). Boxers are taught to push off with their feet in order to move effectively. Forward motion involves lifting the lead leg and pushing with the rear leg. Rearward motion involves lifting the rear leg and pushing with the lead leg. During lateral motion the leg in the direction of the movement moves first while the opposite leg provides the force needed to move the body.

Punches

There are four basic punches in boxing: the jab, cross, hook and uppercut. Any punch other than a jab is considered a power punch. If a boxer is right-handed (orthodox), his left hand is the lead hand and his right hand is the rear hand. For a left-handed boxer or southpaw, the hand positions are reversed. For clarity, the following discussion will assume a right-handed boxer.

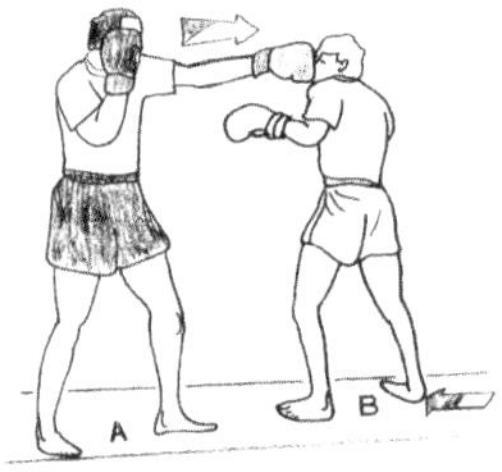

Jab

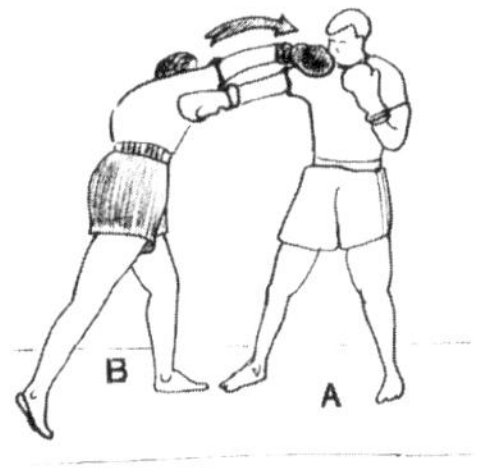

Cross - in counter-punch with a looping

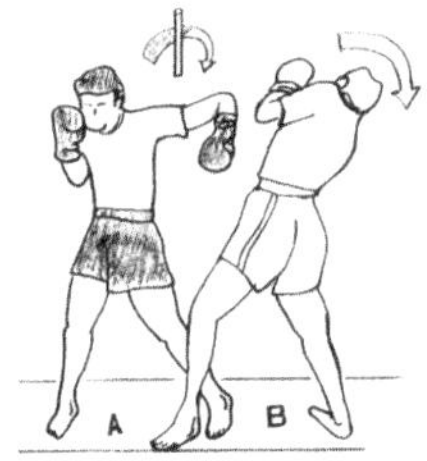

Hook

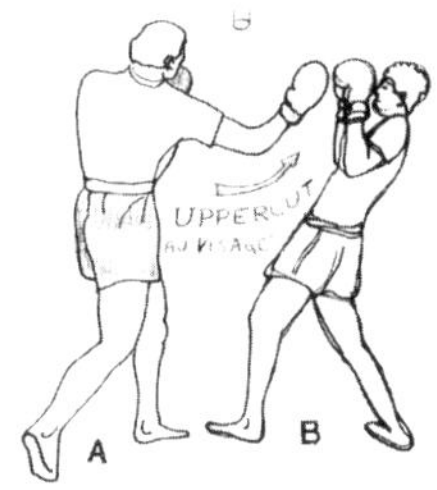

Uppercut

- Jab – A quick, straight punch thrown with the lead hand from the guard position. The jab is accompanied by a small, clockwise rotation of the torso and hips, while the fist rotates 90 degrees, becoming horizontal upon impact. As the punch reaches full extension, the lead shoulder can be brought up to guard the chin. The rear hand remains next to the face to guard the jaw. After making contact with the target, the lead hand is retracted quickly to resume a guard position in front of the face.
    - ◇ The jab is recognized as the most important punch in a boxer's arsenal because it provides a fair amount of its own cover and it leaves the least amount of space for a counter punch from the opponent. It has the longest reach of any punch and does not require commitment or large weight transfers. Due to its relatively weak power, the jab is often used as a tool to gauge distances, probe an opponent's defenses, harass an opponent, and set up heavier, more powerful punches. A half-step may be added, moving the entire body into the punch, for additional power. Some notable boxers who have been able to develop relative power in their jabs and use it to punish or 'wear down' their opponents to some effect include Larry Holmes and Wladimir Klitschko.
- Cross – A powerful, straight punch thrown with the rear hand. From the guard position, the rear hand is thrown from the chin, crossing the body and traveling towards the target in a straight line. The rear shoulder is thrust forward and finishes just touching the outside of the chin. At the same time, the lead hand is retracted and tucked against the face to protect the inside of the chin. For additional power, the torso and hips are rotated counter-clockwise as the cross is thrown. A measure of an ideally extended cross is that the shoulder of the striking arm, the knee of the front leg and the ball of the front foot are on the same vertical plane.
    - ◇ Weight is also transferred from the rear foot to the lead foot, resulting in the rear heel turning outwards as it acts as a fulcrum for the transfer of weight. Body rotation and the sudden weight transfer is what gives the cross its power. Like the jab, a half-step forward may be added. After the cross is thrown, the hand is retracted quickly and the guard position resumed. It can be used to counter punch a jab, aiming for the opponent's head (or a counter to a cross aimed at the body) or to set up a hook. The cross is also called a "straight" or "right", especially if it does not cross the opponent's outstretched jab.
- Hook – A semi-circular punch thrown with the lead hand to the side of the opponent's head. From the guard position, the elbow is drawn back with a horizontal fist (palm facing down) though in modern times a wide percentage of fighters throw the hook with a vertical

fist (palm facing themselves). The rear hand is tucked firmly against the jaw to protect the chin. The torso and hips are rotated clockwise, propelling the fist through a tight, clockwise arc across the front of the body and connecting with the target.

- ◇ At the same time, the lead foot pivots clockwise, turning the left heel outwards. Upon contact, the hook's circular path ends abruptly and the lead hand is pulled quickly back into the guard position. A hook may also target the lower body and this technique is sometimes called the "rip" to distinguish it from the conventional hook to the head. The hook may also be thrown with the rear hand. Notable left hookers include Joe Frazier, Roy Jones Jr. and Mike Tyson.

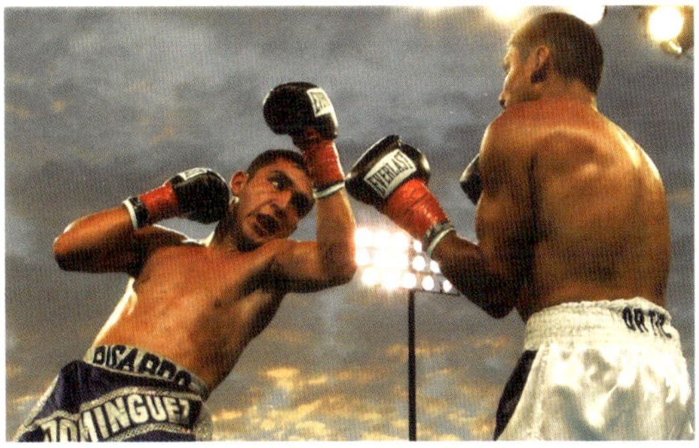

A boxer throws an uppercut.

- Uppercut – A vertical, rising punch thrown with the rear hand. From the guard position, the torso shifts slightly to the right, the rear hand drops below the level of the opponent's chest and the knees are bent slightly. From this position, the rear hand is thrust upwards in a rising arc towards the opponent's chin or torso.
  - ◇ At the same time, the knees push upwards quickly and the torso and hips rotate anti-clockwise and the rear heel turns outward, mimicking the body movement of the cross. The strategic utility of the uppercut depends on its ability to "lift" the opponent's body, setting it off-balance for successive attacks. The right uppercut followed by a left hook is a deadly combination employing the uppercut to lift the opponent's chin into a vulnerable position, then the hook to knock the opponent out.

These different punch types can be thrown in rapid succession to form combinations or "combos." The most common is the jab and cross combination, nicknamed the "one-two combo." This is usually an effective combination, because the jab blocks the opponent's view of the cross, making it easier to land cleanly and forcefully.

A large, swinging circular punch starting from a cocked-back position with the arm at a longer extension than the hook and all of the fighter's weight behind it is sometimes referred to as a "roundhouse," "haymaker," "overhand," or sucker-punch. Relying on body weight and centripetal force within a wide arc, the roundhouse can be a powerful blow, but it is often a wild and uncontrolled punch that leaves the fighter delivering it off balance and with an open guard.

Wide, looping punches have the further disadvantage of taking more time to deliver, giving the opponent ample warning to react and counter. For this reason, the haymaker or roundhouse is not a conventional punch, and is regarded by trainers as a mark of poor technique or desperation.

Sometimes it has been used, because of its immense potential power, to finish off an already staggering opponent who seems unable or unlikely to take advantage of the poor position it leaves the puncher in.

Another unconventional punch is the rarely used bolo punch, in which the opponent swings an arm out several times in a wide arc, usually as a distraction, before delivering with either that or the other arm.

An illegal punch to the back of the head or neck is known as a rabbit punch.

Both the hook and uppercut may be thrown with both hands, resulting in differing footwork and positioning from that described above if thrown by the other hand. Generally the analogous opposite is true of the footwork and torso movement.

Defense

There are several basic maneuvers a boxer can use in order to evade or block punches, depicted and discussed below.

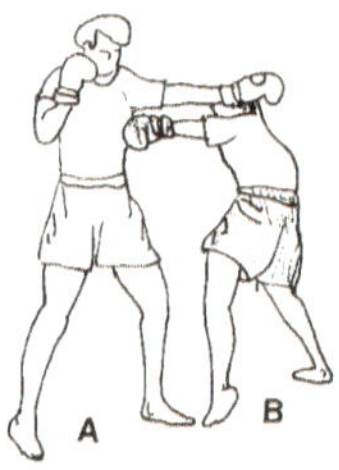

Slipping

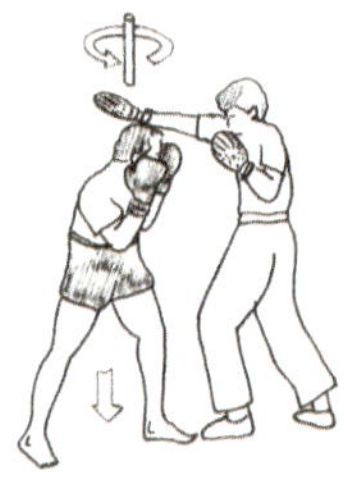

[Bobbing

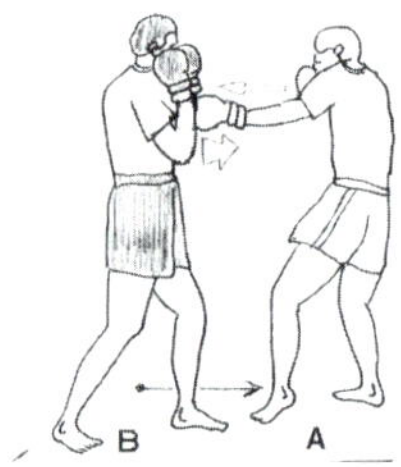

Blocking (with the arms)

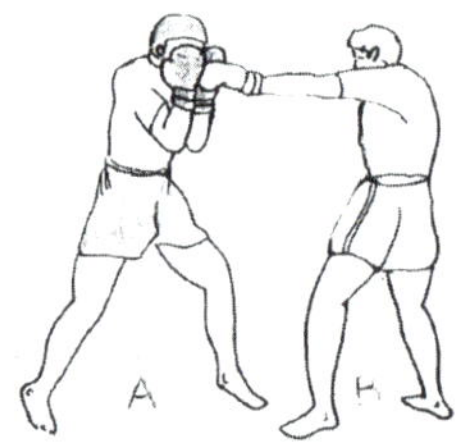

Cover-Up (with the gloves)

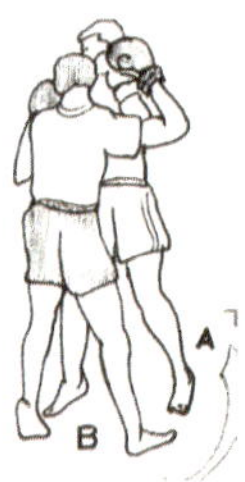

Clinching

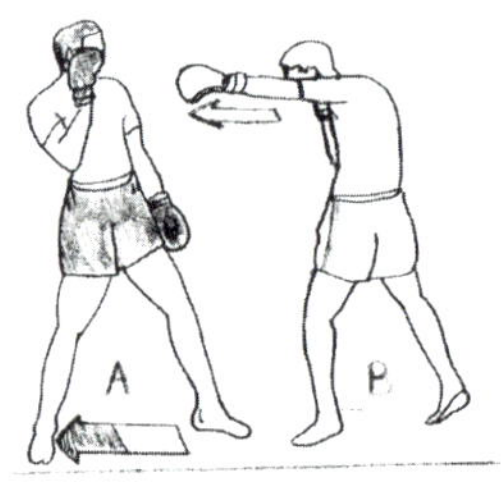

Footwork

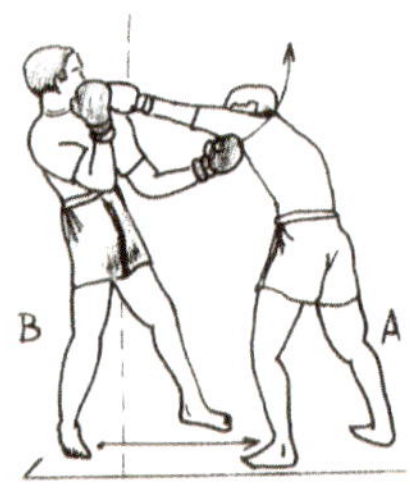

Pulling away

- Slip – Slipping rotates the body slightly so that an incoming punch passes harmlessly next to the head. As the opponent's punch arrives, the boxer sharply rotates the hips and shoulders. This turns the chin sideways and allows the punch to "slip" past. Muhammad Ali was famous for extremely fast and close slips, as was an early Mike Tyson.
- Sway or fade – To anticipate a punch and move the upper body or head back so that it misses or has its force appreciably lessened. Also called "rolling with the punch" or " Riding The Punch".
- Duck or break – To drop down with the back straight so that a punch aimed at the head glances or misses entirely.

- Bob and weave – Bobbing moves the head laterally and beneath an incoming punch. As the opponent's punch arrives, the boxer bends the legs quickly and simultaneously shifts the body either slightly right or left. Once the punch has been evaded, the boxer "weaves" back to an upright position, emerging on either the outside or inside of the opponent's still-extended arm. To move outside the opponent's extended arm is called "bobbing to the outside". To move inside the opponent's extended arm is called "bobbing to the inside". Joe Frazier, Jack Dempsey, Mike Tyson and Rocky Marciano were masters of bobbing and weaving.
- Parry/block – Parrying or blocking uses the boxer's shoulder, hands or arms as defensive tools to protect against incoming attacks. A block generally receives a punch while a parry tends to deflect it. A "palm", "catch", or "cuff" is a defence which intentionally takes the incoming punch on the palm portion of the defender's glove.
- The cover-up – Covering up is the last opportunity (other than rolling with a punch) to avoid an incoming strike to an unprotected face or body. Generally speaking, the hands are held high to protect the head and chin and the forearms are tucked against the torso to impede body shots. When protecting the body, the boxer rotates the hips and lets incoming punches "roll" off the guard. To protect the head, the boxer presses both fists against the front of the face with the forearms parallel and facing outwards. This type of guard is weak against attacks from below.
- The clinch – Clinching is a form of trapping or a rough form of grappling and occurs when the distance between both fighters has closed and straight punches cannot be employed. In this situation, the boxer attempts to hold or "tie up" the opponent's hands so he is unable to throw hooks or uppercuts. To perform a clinch, the boxer loops both hands around the outside of the opponent's shoulders, scooping back under the forearms to grasp the opponent's arms tightly against his own body. In this position, the opponent's arms are pinned and cannot be used to attack. Clinching is a temporary match state and is quickly dissipated by the referee. Clinching is technically against the rules, and in amateur fights points are deducted fairly quickly for it. It is unlikely, however, to see points deducted for a clinch in professional boxing.

Less Common Strategies

- The "rope-a-dope" strategy : Used by Muhammad Ali in his 1974 "the Rumble in the Jungle" bout against George Foreman, the rope-a-dope method involves lying back against the ropes, covering up defensively as much as possible and allowing the opponent to attempt numerous punches. The back-leaning posture, which does not cause the defending boxer to become as unbalanced as he would during normal backward movement, also maximizes the distance of the defender's head from his opponent, increasing the probability that punches will miss their intended target. Weathering the blows that do land, the defender lures the opponent into expending energy while conserving his/her own. If successful, the attacking opponent will eventually tire, creating defensive flaws which the boxer can exploit. In modern boxing, the rope-a-dope is generally discouraged since most opponents are not fooled by it and few boxers possess the physical toughness to withstand a prolonged, unanswered assault. Recently, however, eight-division world champion Manny Pacquiao skillfully used the strategy to gauge the power of welterweight titlist Miguel Cotto in November 2009. Pacquiao followed up the rope-a-dope gambit with a withering knockdown.

- Bolo punch : Occasionally seen in Olympic boxing, the bolo is an arm punch which owes its power to the shortening of a circular arc rather than to transference of body weight; it tends to have more of an effect due to the surprise of the odd angle it lands at rather than the actual power of the punch. This is more of a gimmick than a technical maneuver; this punch is not taught, being on the same plane in boxing technicality as is the Ali shuffle. Nevertheless, a few professional boxers have used the bolo-punch to great effect, including former welterweight champions Sugar Ray Leonard, and Kid Gavilan. Middleweight champion Ceferino Garcia is regarded as the inventor of the bolo punch.

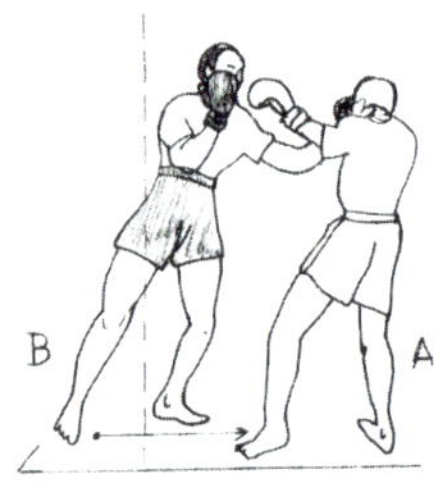

Bolo punch

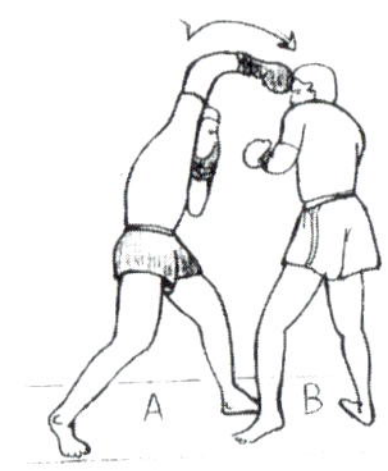

Overhand (overcut)

- Overhand right : The overhand right is a punch not found in every boxer's arsenal. Unlike the right cross, which has a trajectory parallel to the ground, the overhand right has a looping circular arc as it is thrown over the shoulder with the palm facing away from the boxer. It is especially popular with smaller stature boxers trying to reach taller opponents. Boxers who have used this punch consistently and effectively include former heavyweight champions Rocky Marciano and Tim Witherspoon, as well as MMA champions Chuck Liddell and Fedor Emelianenko. The overhand right has become a popular weapon in other tournaments that involve fist striking.

- Check hook : A check hook is employed to prevent aggressive boxers from lunging in. There are two parts to the check hook. The first part consists of a regular hook. The second, trickier part involves the footwork. As the opponent lunges in, the boxer should throw the hook and pivot on his left foot and swing his right foot 180 degrees around. If executed correctly, the aggressive boxer will lunge in and sail harmlessly past his opponent like a bull missing a matador. This is rarely seen in professional boxing as it requires a great disparity in skill level to execute. Technically speaking it has been said that there is no such thing as a check hook and that it is simply a hook applied to an opponent that has lurched forward and past his opponent who simply hooks him on the way past. Others have argued that the check hook exists but is an illegal punch due to it being a pivot punch which is illegal in the sport. Floyd Mayweather, Jr. employed the use of a check hook against Ricky Hatton, which sent Hatton flying head first into the corner post and being knocked down.

Ring Corner

In boxing, each fighter is given a corner of the ring where he rests in between rounds for 1 minute and where his trainers stand. Typically, three men stand in the corner besides the boxer himself; these are the trainer, the assistant trainer and the cutman. The trainer and assistant typically give advice to the boxer on what he is doing wrong as well as encouraging him if he is losing. The cutman is a cutaneous doctor responsible for keeping the boxer's face and eyes free of cuts and blood. This is of particular importance because many fights are stopped because of cuts that threaten the boxer's eyes.

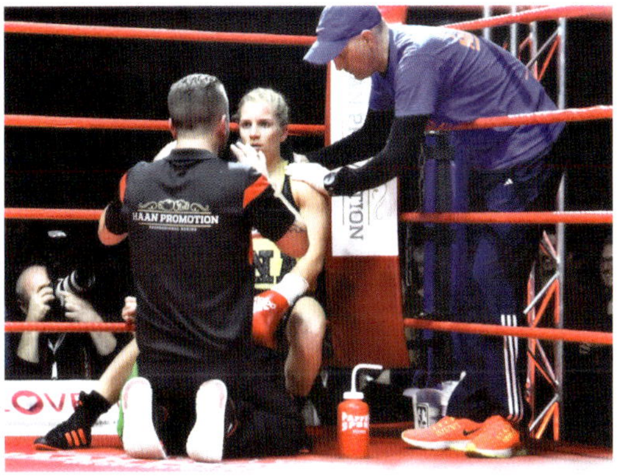

A female boxer receiving instructions from her trainer while being treated by her cutman in the ring corner between rounds.

In addition, the corner is responsible for stopping the fight if they feel their fighter is in grave danger of permanent injury. The corner will occasionally throw in a white towel to signify a boxer's surrender (the idiomatic phrase "to throw in the towel", meaning to give up, derives from this practice). This can be seen in the fight between Diego Corrales and Floyd Mayweather. In that fight, Corrales' corner surrendered despite Corrales' steadfast refusal.

Medical Concerns

Knocking a person unconscious or even causing a concussion may cause permanent brain damage. There is no clear division between the force required to knock a person out and the force likely to kill a person. From 1980 to 2007, more than 200 amateur boxers, professional boxers and Toughman fighters died due to ring or training injuries. The editor, Dr. George Lundberg, called boxing an "obscenity" that "should not be sanctioned by any civilized society." Since then, the British, Canadian and Australian Medical Associations have called for bans on boxing.

Supporters of the ban state that boxing is the only sport where hurting the other athlete is the goal. Dr. Bill O'Neill, boxing spokesman for the British Medical Association, has supported the BMA's proposed ban on boxing: "It is the only sport where the intention is to inflict serious injury on your opponent, and we feel that we must have a total ban on boxing." Opponents respond that such a position is misguided opinion, stating that amateur boxing is scored solely according to total connecting blows with no award for "injury". They observe that many skilled professional boxers have had rewarding careers without inflicting injury on opponents by accumulating scoring blows and avoiding punches winning rounds scored 10-9 by the 10-point must system, and they note that there are many other sports where concussions are much more prevalent.

In 2007, one study of amateur boxers showed that protective headgear did not prevent brain damage, and another found that amateur boxers faced a high risk of brain damage. The Gothenburg study analyzed temporary levels of neurofiliment light in cerebral spinal fluid which they conclude is evidence of damage, even though the levels soon subside. More comprehensive studies of neurologiocal function on larger samples performed by Johns Hopkins University and accident rates analyzed by National Safety Council show amateur boxing is a comparatively safe sport.

In 1997, the American Association of Professional Ringside Physicians was established to create medical protocols through research and education to prevent injuries in boxing.

Professional boxing is forbidden in Iceland, Iran, Saudi Arabia and North Korea. It was banned in Sweden until 2007 when the ban was lifted but strict restrictions, including four three-minute rounds for fights, were imposed. It was banned in Albania from 1965 till the fall of Communism in 1991; it is now legal there. Norway legalized professional boxing in December 2014.

Boxing Hall of Fame

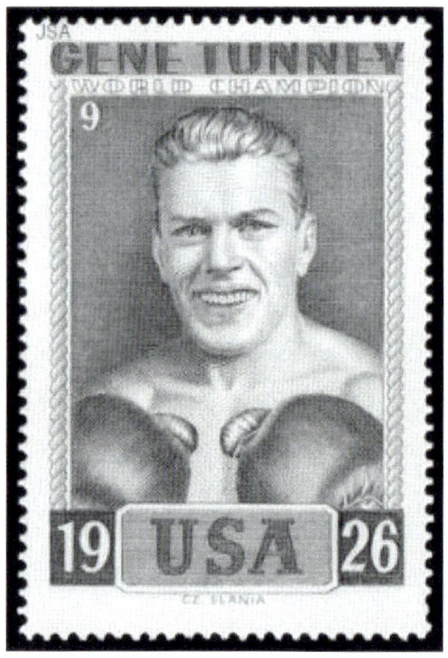

Stamp honoring heavyweight champion.

The sport of boxing has two internationally recognized boxing halls of fame; the International Boxing Hall of Fame (IBHOF) and the World Boxing Hall of Fame (WBHF), with the IBHOF being the more widely recognized boxing hall of fame. In 2013, The Boxing Hall of Fame Las Vegas opened in Las Vegas, NV founded by Steve Lott, former assistant manager for Mike Tyson.

The WBHF was founded by Everett L. Sanders in 1980. Since its inception, the WBHOF has never had a permanent location or museum, which has allowed the more recent IBHOF to garner more publicity and prestige. Among the notable names in the WBHF are Ricardo "Finito" Lopez, Gabriel "Flash" Elorde, Michael Carbajal, Khaosai Galaxy, Henry Armstrong, Jack Johnson, Roberto Durán, George Foreman, Ceferino Garcia and Salvador Sanchez. Boxing's International Hall of Fame was inspired by a tribute an American town held for two local heroes in 1982. The town, Canastota, New York, (which is about 15 miles (24 km) east of Syracuse, via the New York State Thruway), honored former world welterweight/middleweight champion Carmen Basilio and his nephew, former world welterweight champion Billy Backus. The people of Canastota raised money for the tribute which inspired the idea of creating an official, annual hall of fame for notable boxers.

The International Boxing Hall of Fame opened in Canastota in 1989. The first inductees in 1990 included Jack Johnson, Benny Leonard, Jack Dempsey, Henry Armstrong, Sugar Ray Robinson,

Archie Moore, and Muhammad Ali. Other world-class figures include Salvador Sanchez, Jose Napoles, Roberto “Manos de Piedra” Durán, Ricardo Lopez, Gabriel “Flash” Elorde, Vicente Saldivar, Ismael Laguna, Eusebio Pedroza, Carlos Monzón, Azumah Nelson, Rocky Marciano, Pipino Cuevas and Ken Buchanan. The Hall of Fame’s induction ceremony is held every June as part of a four-day event. The fans who come to Canastota for the Induction Weekend are treated to a number of events, including scheduled autograph sessions, boxing exhibitions, a parade featuring past and present inductees, and the induction ceremony itself.

The Boxing Hall of Fame Las Vegas features the $75 million ESPN Classic Sports fight film and tape library and radio broadcast collection. The collection includes the fights of all the great champions including: Muhammad Ali, Mike Tyson, George Foreman, Roberto Duran, Marvin Hagler, Jack Dempsey, Joe Louis, Joe Frazier, Rocky Marciano and Sugar Ray Robinson. It is this exclusive fight film library that will separate the Boxing Hall of Fame Las Vegas from the other halls of fame which do not have rights to any video of their sports. The inaugural inductees included Muhammad Ali, Henry Armstrong, Tony Canzoneri, Ezzard Charles, Julio César Chávez Sr., Jack Dempsey, Roberto Duran, Joe Louis, and Sugar Ray Robinson

Walking

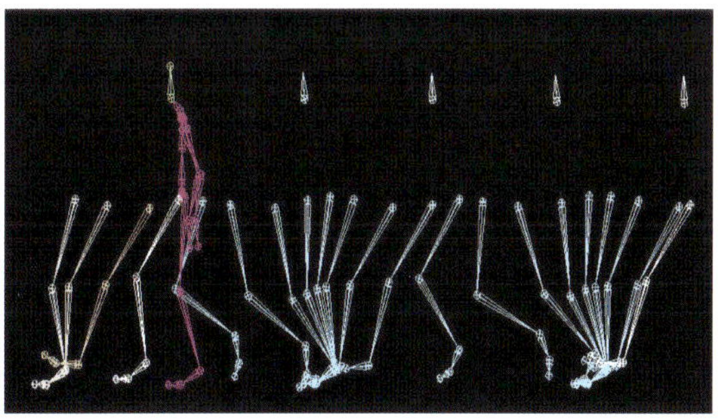

Computer simulation of a human walk cycle. In this model the head keeps the same level at all times, whereas the hip follows a sine curve.

Walking (also known as ambulation) is one of the main gaits of locomotion among legged animals. Walking is typically slower than running and other gaits. Walking is defined by an ‘inverted pendulum’ gait in which the body vaults over the stiff limb or limbs with each step. This applies regardless of the number of limbs—even arthropods, with six, eight or more limbs, walk.

Difference from Running

The word *walk* is descended from the Old English *wealcan* “to roll”. In humans and other bipeds, walking is generally distinguished from running in that only one foot at a time leaves contact with the ground and there is a period of double-support. In contrast, running begins when both feet are off the ground with each step. This distinction has the status of a formal requirement in competitive walking events. For quadrupedal species, there are numerous gaits which may be termed walking or running, and distinctions based upon the presence or absence of a suspended phase or the number of feet in contact any time do not yield mechanically correct classification. The most effective method to distinguish walking from running is to measure the height of a person’s centre of mass using motion capture or a force plate at midstance. During walking, the centre of mass reaches a maximum height at midstance, while during running, it is then at a minimum. This distinction, however, only holds true for locomotion over level or approximately level ground. For walking up grades above 10%, this distinction no longer holds for some individuals. Definitions based on the percentage of the stride during which a foot is in contact with the ground (averaged across all feet) of greater than 50% contact corresponds well with identification of 'inverted pendulum' mechanics and are indicative of walking for animals with any number of limbs, although this definition is incomplete. Running humans and animals may have contact periods greater than 50% of a gait cycle when rounding corners, running uphill or carrying loads.

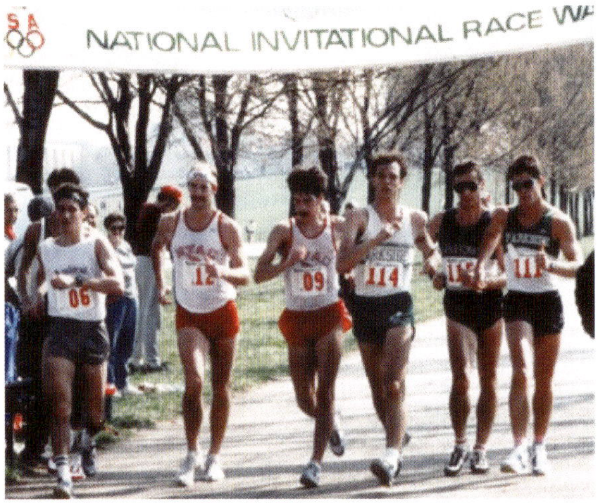

Racewalkers at the World Cup Trials.

Speed is another factor that distinguishes walking from running. Although walking speeds can vary greatly depending on many factors such as height, weight, age, terrain, surface, load, culture, effort, and fitness, the average human walking speed at crosswalks is about 5.0 kilometres per hour (km/h), or about 1.4 meters per second (m/s), or about 3.1 miles per hour (mph). Specific studies have found pedestrian walking speeds at crosswalks ranging from 4.51 kilometres per hour (2.80 mph) to 4.75 kilometres per hour (2.95 mph) for older individuals and from 5.32 kilometres per hour (3.31 mph) to 5.43 kilometres per hour (3.37 mph) for younger individuals; a brisk walking speed can be around 6.5 kilometres per hour (4.0 mph). Champion racewalkers can average more than 14 kilometres per hour (8.7 mph) over a distance of 20 kilometres (12 mi).

An average human child achieves independent walking ability at around 11 months old.

Health Benefits

Regular, brisk exercise of any kind can improve confidence, stamina, energy, weight control and life expectancy and reduce stress. It can also reduce the risk of coronary heart disease, strokes, diabetes, high blood pressure, bowel cancer and osteoporosis. Scientific studies have also shown that walking, besides its physical benefits, is also beneficial for the mind, improving memory skills, learning ability, concentration and abstract reasoning, as well as ameliorating spirits. Sustained walking sessions for a minimum period of thirty to sixty minutes a day, five days a week, with the correct walking posture, reduce health risks and have various overall health benefits, such as reducing the chances of cancer, type 2 diabetes, heart disease, anxiety disorder and depression. Life expectancy is also increased even for individuals suffering from obesity or high blood pressure. Walking also improves bone health, especially strengthening the hip bone, and lowering the harmful low-density lipoprotein (LDL) cholesterol, and raising the useful high-density lipoprotein (HDL) cholesterol. Studies have found that walking may also help prevent dementia and Alzheimer's.

The Centers for Disease Control and Prevention's fact sheet on the "Relationship of Walking to Mortality Among U.S. Adults with Diabetes" states that those with diabetes who walked for 2 or more hours a week lowered their mortality rate from all causes by 39 per cent. "Walking lengthened the life of people with diabetes regardless of age, sex, race, body mass index, length of time since diagnosis, and presence of complications or functional limitations." It has been suggested that there is a relationship between the speed of walking and health, and that the best results are obtained with a speed of more than 2.5 mph (4 km/h).

Governments now recognize the benefits of walking for mental and physical health and are actively encouraging it. This growing emphasis on walking has arisen because people walk less nowadays than previously. In the UK, a Department of Transport report found that between 1995/97 and 2005 the average number of walk trips per person fell by 16%, from 292 to 245 per year. Many professionals in local authorities and the NHS are employed to halt this decline by ensuring that the built environment allows people to walk and that there are walking opportunities available to them. Professionals working to encourage walking come mainly from six sectors: health, transport, environment, schools, sport and recreation, and urban design.

One programme to encourage walking is "The Walking the Way to Health Initiative", organized by the British walkers association The Ramblers, which is the largest volunteer led walking scheme in the United Kingdom. Volunteers are trained to lead free Health Walks from community venues such as libraries and doctors' surgeries. The scheme has trained over 35,000 volunteers and have over 500 schemes operating across the UK, with thousands of people walking every week. A new organization called "Walk England" launched a web site in June 2008 to provide these professionals with evidence, advice and examples of success stories of how to encourage communities to walk more. The site has a social networking aspect to allow professionals and the public to ask questions, post news and events and communicate with others in their area about walking, as well as a "walk now" option to find out what walks are available in each region. Similar organizations exist in other countries and recently a "Walking Summit" was held in the United States. This "assembl[ed] thought-leaders and influencers from business, urban planning and real estate, [along with] physicians and public health officials," and others, to discuss how to make American cities and communities places where "people can and want to walk".

Origins

It is theorized that "walking" among tetrapods originated underwater with air-breathing fish that could "walk" underwater, giving rise to the plethora of land-dwelling life that walk on four or two limbs. While terrestrial tetrapods are theorised to have a single origin, arthropods and their relatives are thought to have independently evolved walking several times, specifically in insects, myriapods, chelicerates, tardigrades, onychophorans, and crustaceans. Little skates, members of the demersal fish community, can propel themselves by pushing off the ocean floor with their pelvic fins, using neural mechanisms which evolved as early as 420 million years ago, before vertebrates set foot on land.,

Judging from footprints discovered on a former shore in Kenya, it is thought possible that ancestors of modern humans were walking in ways very similar to the present activity as many as 1.5 million years ago.

Variants

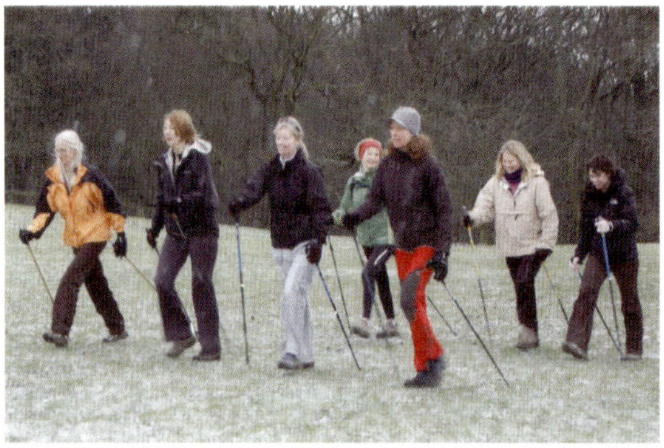

Nordic walkers.

- Scrambling is a method of ascending a hill or mountain that involves using both hands, because of the steepness of the terrain. Of necessity it will be a slow and careful form of walking and with possibly of occasional brief, easy rock climbing. Some scrambling takes place on narrow exposed ridges where more attention to balance will be required than in normal walking.

- Snow shoeing – A snowshoe is footwear for walking over the snow. Snowshoes work by distributing the weight of the person over a larger area so that the person's foot does not sink completely into the snow, a quality called "flotation". It is often said by snowshoers that if you can walk, you can snowshoe. This is true in optimal conditions, but snowshoeing properly requires some slight adjustments to walking. The method of walking is to lift the shoes slightly and slide the inner edges over each other, thus avoiding the unnatural and fatiguing "straddle-gait" that would otherwise be necessary. A snowshoer must be willing to roll his or her feet slightly as well. An exaggerated stride works best when starting out, particularly with larger or traditional shoes.

- Beach walking is a sport that is based on walk on the sand of the beach. Beach walking can be developed on compact sand or non-compact sand. There are beach walking competitions on non-compact sand. And there are world records of beach walking on non-compact sand in Multiday distances. Beach walking has a specific technique of walk.

- Nordic walking is a physical activity and a sport, which is performed with specially designed walking poles similar to ski poles. Compared to regular walking, Nordic walking (also called pole walking) involves applying force to the poles with each stride. Nordic walkers use more of their entire body (with greater intensity) and receive fitness building stimulation not present in normal walking for the chest, lats, triceps, biceps, shoulder, abdominals, spinal and other core muscles that may result in significant increases in heart rate at a given pace. Nordic walking has been estimated as producing up to a 46% increase in energy consumption, compared to walking without poles.

- Pedestrianism is a sport that developed during the late eighteenth and nineteenth centuries, and was a popular spectator sport in the British Isles. By the end of the 18th century, and especially with the growth of the popular press, feats of foot travel over great distances (similar to a modern ultramarathon) gained attention, and were labeled "pedestrianism". Interest in the sport, and the wagering which accompanied it, spread to the United States, Canada, and Australia in the 19th century. By the end of the 19th century, Pedestrianism was largely displaced by the rise in modern spectator sports and by controversy involving rules, which limited its appeal as a source of wagering and led to its inclusion in the amateur athletics movement. Pedestrianism was first codified in the last half of the 19th century, evolving into what would become racewalking, By the mid 19th century, competitors were often expected to extend their legs straight at least once in their stride, and obey what was called the "fair heel and toe" rule. This rule, the source of modern racewalking, was a vague commandment that the toe of one foot could not leave the ground before the heel of the next foot touched down. This said, rules were customary and changed with competition. Racers were usually allowed to jog in order to fend off cramps, and it was distance, not code, which determined gait for longer races. Newspaper reports suggest that "trotting" was common in events.

- Power walking or speed walking is the act of walking with a speed at the upper end of the natural range for walking gait, typically 7 to 9 km/h (4.5 to 5.5 mph). To qualify as power walking as opposed to jogging or running, at least one foot must be in contact with the ground at all times.

- Racewalking is a long-distance athletic event. Although it is a foot race, it is different from running in that one foot must appear to be in contact with the ground at all times. Stride length is reduced, so to achieve competitive speeds, racewalkers must attain cadence rates comparable to those achieved by Olympic 800-meter runners, and they must do so for hours at a time since the Olympic events are the 20 km (12.4 mi) race walk (men and women) and 50 km (31 mi) race walk (men only), and 50 mile (80.5 km) events are also held.

- Afghan walking: The Afghan Walk is a rhythmic breathing technique synchronized with walking. It was born in the 1980s on the basis of the observations made by the Frenchman Édouard G. Stiegler, during his contacts with Afghan caravaners, capable of making walks of more than 60 km per day for dozens of days.

Biomechanics

Human walking is accomplished with a strategy called the double pendulum. During forward motion, the leg that leaves the ground swings forward from the hip. This sweep is the first pendulum. Then the leg strikes the ground with the heel and rolls through to the toe in a motion described as an inverted pendulum. The motion of the two legs is coordinated so that one foot or the other is always in contact with the ground. The process of walking recovers approximately sixty per cent of the energy used due to pendulum dynamics and ground reaction force.

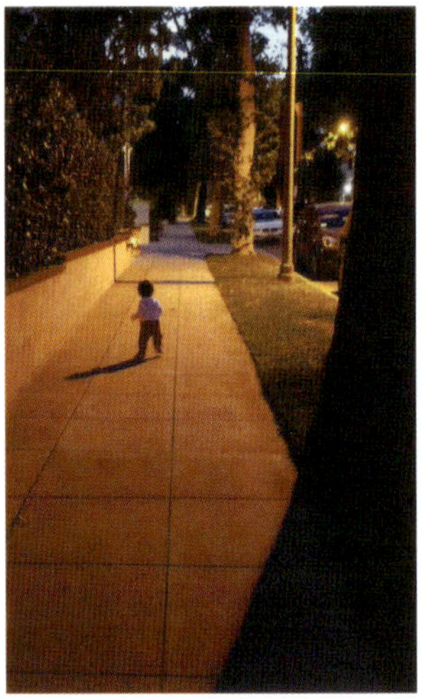

Young child walking on a street

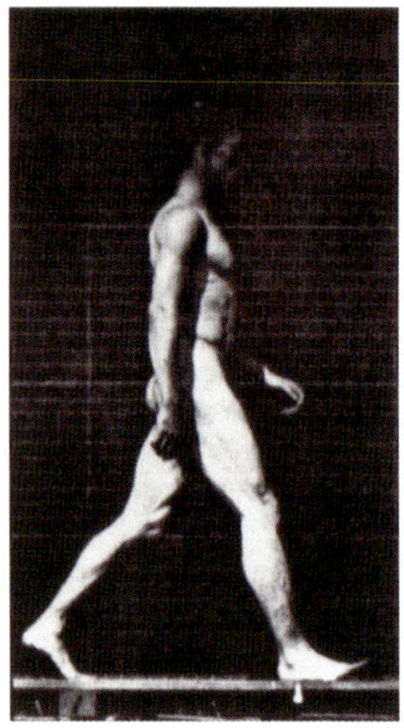

Human Walking Cycle

Walking differs from a running gait in a number of ways. The most obvious is that during walking one leg always stays on the ground while the other is swinging. In running there is typically a ballistic phase where the runner is airborne with both feet in the air (for bipedals).

Another difference concerns the movement of the centre of mass of the body. In walking the body "vaults" over the leg on the ground, raising the centre of mass to its highest point as the leg passes the vertical, and dropping it to the lowest as the legs are spread apart. Essentially kinetic energy of forward motion is constantly being traded for a rise in potential energy. This is reversed in running where the centre of mass is at its lowest as the leg is vertical. This is because the impact of landing from the ballistic phase is absorbed by bending the leg and consequently storing energy in muscles and tendons. In running there is a conversion between kinetic, potential, and elastic energy.

There is an absolute limit on an individual's speed of walking (without special techniques such as those employed in speed walking) due to the upwards acceleration of the centre of mass during a stride – if it's greater than the acceleration due to gravity the person will become airborne as they vault over the leg on the ground. Typically however, animals switch to a run at a lower speed than this due to energy efficiencies.

Based on the 2D inverted pendulum model of walking, there are at least five physical constraints that place fundamental limits on walking like an inverted pendulum. These constraints are: take-off constraint, sliding constraint, fall-back constraint, steady-state constraint, high step-frequency constraint.

A Leisure Activity

Many people enjoy walking as a recreation in the mainly urban modern world, and it is one of the best forms of exercise. For some, walking is a way to enjoy nature and the outdoors; and for others the physical, sporting and endurance aspect is more important.

There are a variety of different kinds of walking, including bushwalking, racewalking, beach walking, hillwalking, volksmarching, Nordic walking, trekking and hiking. Some people prefer to walk indoors on a treadmill, or in a gym, and fitness walkers and others may use a pedometer to count their steps. Hiking is the usual word used in Canada, the United States and South Africa for long vigorous walks; similar walks are called tramps in New Zealand, or hill walking or just walking in Australia, the UK and the Irish Republic. Australians also bushwalk. In English-speaking parts of North America the term walking is used for short walks, especially in towns and cities. Snow shoeing is walking in snow; a slightly different gait is required compared with regular walking.

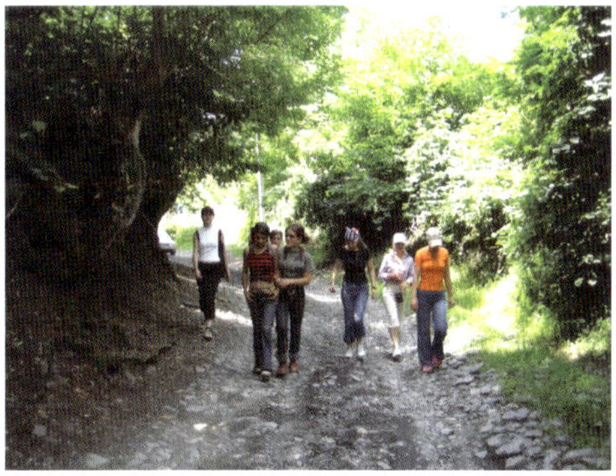

Walking in Shilda, Georgia.

In terms of tourism the possibilities range from guided walking tours in cities, to organized trekking holidays in the Himalayas. In the UK the term walking tour also refers to a multi-day walk or hike undertaken by a group or individual. Well-organized systems of trails exist in many other European counties, as well as Canada, United States, New Zealand, and Nepal. Systems of lengthy waymarked walking trails now stretch across Europe from Norway to Turkey, Portugal to Cyprus. Many also walk the traditional pilgrim routes, of which the most famous is El Camino de Santiago, The Way of St. James.

Numerous walking festivals and other walking events take place each year in many countries. The world's largest multi-day walking event is the International Four Days Marches Nijmegen in the Netherlands. The "Vierdaagse" (Dutch for "Four day Event") is an annual walk that has taken place since 1909; it has been based at Nijmegen since 1916. Depending on age group and category, walkers have to walk 30, 40 or 50 kilometers each day for four days. Originally a military event with a few civilians, it now is a mainly civilian event. Numbers have risen in recent years, with over 40,000 now taking part, including about 5,000 military personnel. Due to crowds on the route, since 2004 the organizers have limited the number of participants. In the U.S., there is the annual Labor Day walk on Mackinac Bridge, Michigan, which draws over 60,000 participants; it is the largest single-day walking event; while the Chesapeake Bay Bridge Walk in Maryland draws over 50,000 participants each year. There are also various walks organised as charity events, with walkers sponsored for a specific cause. These walks range in length from two miles (3 km) or five km to 50 miles (80 km). The MS Challenge Walk is an 80 km or 50 mile walk which raises money to fight multiple sclerosis, while walkers in the Oxfam Trailwalker cover 100 km or 60 miles.

In Britain, The Ramblers, a registered charity, is the largest organisation that looks after the interests of walkers, with some 100,000 members. Its "Get Walking Keep Walking" project provides free route guides, led walks, as well as information for people new to walking. The Long Distance Walkers Association in the UK is for the more energetic walker, and organizes lengthy challenge hikes of 20 or even 50 miles (30 to 80 km) or more in a day. The LDWA's annual "Hundred" event, entailing walking 100 miles or 160 km in 48 hours, takes place each British Spring Bank Holiday weekend.

Walkability

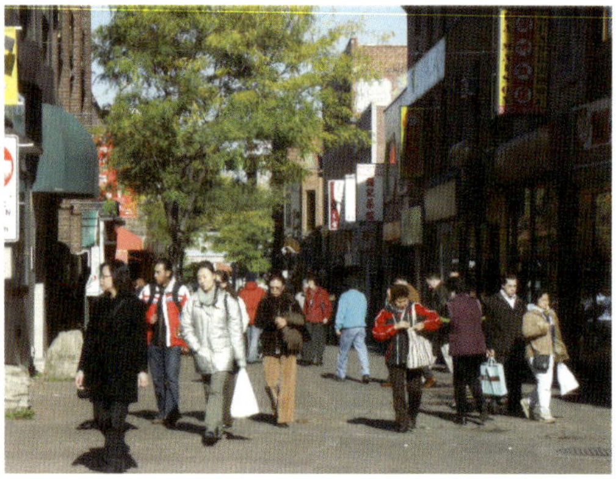

Gauchetière Street, Montreal, Quebec, Canada.

There has been a recent focus among urban planners in some communities to create pedestrian-friendly areas and roads, allowing commuting, shopping and recreation to be done on foot. The concept of walkability has arisen as a measure of the degree to which an area is friendly to walking. Some communities are at least partially car-free, making them particularly supportive of walking and other modes of transportation. In the United States, the active living network is an example of a concerted effort to develop communities more friendly to walking and other physical activities.

An example of such efforts to make urban development more pedestrian friendly is the pedestrian village. This is a compact, pedestrian-oriented neighborhood or town, with a mixed-use village center, that follows the tenets of New Pedestrianism. Shared-use lanes for pedestrians and those using bicycles, Segways, wheelchairs, and other small rolling conveyances that do not use internal combustion engines. Generally, these lanes are in front of the houses and businesses, and streets for motor vehicles are always at the rear. Some pedestrian villages might be nearly car-free with cars either hidden below the buildings or on the periphery of the village. Venice, Italy is essentially a pedestrian village with canals. The canal district in Venice, California, on the other hand, combines the front lane/rear street approach with canals and walkways, or just walkways.

Walking is also considered to be a clear example of a sustainable mode of transport, especially suited for urban use and/or relatively shorter distances. Non-motorised transport modes such as walking, but also cycling, small-wheeled transport (skates, skateboards, push scooters and hand carts) or wheelchair travel are often key elements of successfully encouraging clean urban transport. A large variety of case studies and good practices (from European cities and some worldwide examples) that promote and stimulate walking as a means of transportation in cities can be found at Eltis, Europe's portal for local transport.

The development of specific rights of way with appropriate infrastructure can promote increased participation and enjoyment of walking. Examples of types of investment include pedestrian malls, and foreshoreways such as oceanways and also river walks.

The first purpose-built pedestrian street in Europe is the Lijnbaan in Rotterdam, opened in 1953. The first pedestrianised shopping centre in the United Kingdom was in Stevenage in 1959. A large number of European towns and cities have made part of their centres car-free since the early 1960s. These are often accompanied by car parks on the edge of the pedestrianised zone, and, in the larger cases, park and ride schemes. Central Copenhagen is one of the largest and oldest: It was converted from car traffic into pedestrian zone in 1962.

In Robotics

The first successful attempts at walking robots tended to have six legs. The number of legs was reduced as microprocessor technology advanced, and there are now a number of robots that can walk on two legs. One, for example, is ASIMO. Although robots have taken great strides in advancement, they still don't walk nearly as well as human beings as they often need to keep their knees bent permanently in order to improve stability.

In 2009, Japanese roboticist Tomotaka Takahashi developed a robot that can jump three inches off the ground. The robot, named Ropid, is capable of getting up, walking, running, and jumping.

In Child Amputees

Walking for normal able bodied children is a lot different than walking for below-knee-amputees. Walking is less fluid and symmetrical for the children who are amputees. Research was conducted in order to find the best way to get the amputee children to develop a more symmetrical and fluid walking form like normal able bodied children. Because of the results of the study which showed that the normal bodied children can withstand a lot more external loading than the amputees, researchers are now looking into the manufacturing and design of the prosthetics that these amputees use. Potentially, they could come up a new idea or a model that can improve the walking capabilities of these amputee children.

Cycling

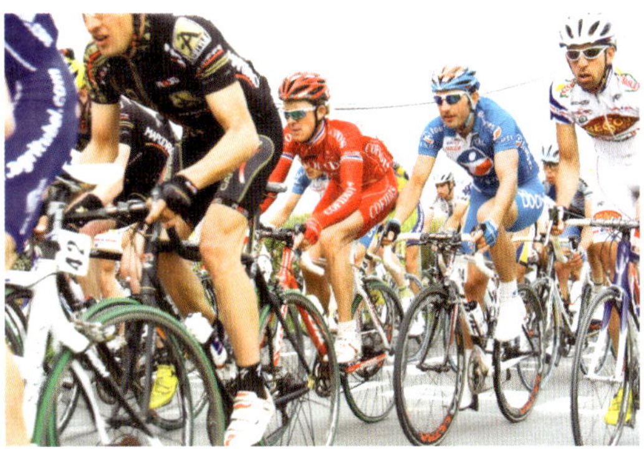

Tro-Bro Léon racing.

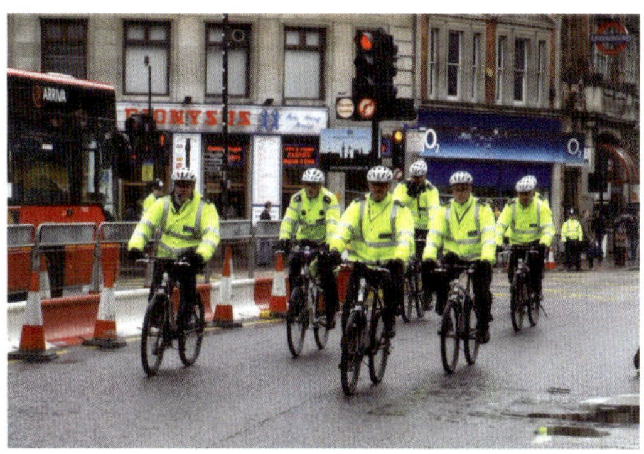

Police cyclists in London.

Cycling, also called bicycling or biking, is the use of bicycles for transport, recreation, exercise or sport. People engaged in cycling are referred to as "cyclists", "bikers", or less commonly, as "bicyclists". Apart from two-wheeled bicycles, "cycling" also includes the riding of unicycles, tricycles, quadracycles, recumbent and similar human-powered vehicles (HPVs).

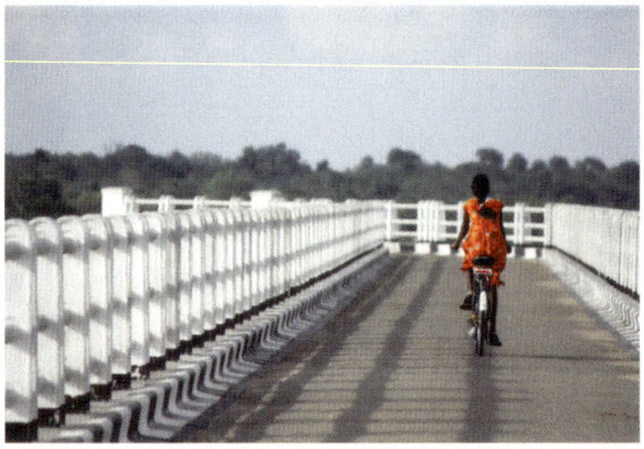

Village cycling in Sri Lanka.

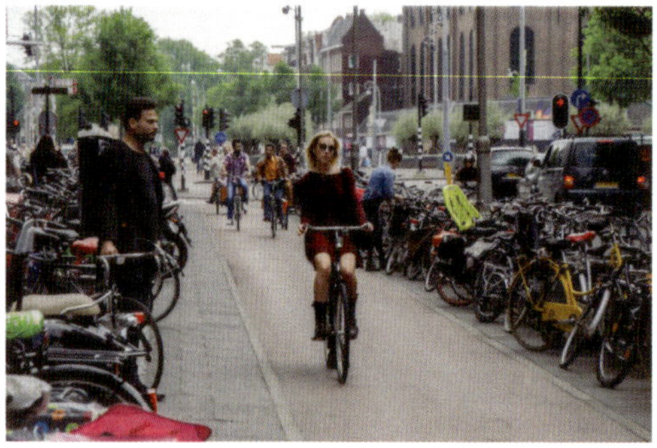

Along the *Fietspad* in Amsterdam, safe from traffic.

Bicycles were introduced in the 19th century and now number approximately one billion worldwide. They are the principal means of transportation in many parts of the world.

Cycling is widely regarded as a very effective and efficient mode of transportation optimal for short to moderate distances.

Bicycles provide numerous benefits in comparison with motor vehicles, including the sustained physical exercise involved in cycling, easier parking, increased maneuverability, and access to roads, bike paths and rural trails. Cycling also offers a reduced consumption of fossil fuels, less air or noise pollution, and much reduced traffic congestion. These lead to less financial cost to the user as well as to society at large (negligible damage to roads, less road area required). By fitting bicycle racks on the front of buses, transit agencies can significantly increase the areas they can serve.

Among the disadvantages of cycling are the requirement of bicycles (excepting tricycles or quadracycles) to be balanced by the rider in order to remain upright, the reduced protection in crashes in comparison to motor vehicles, often longer travel time (except in densely populated areas), vulnerability to weather conditions, difficulty in transporting passengers, and the fact that a basic level of fitness is required for cycling moderate to long distances.

Equipment

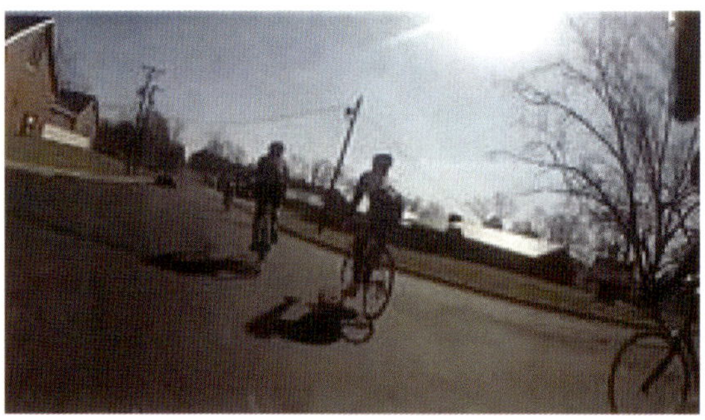

Cycling in Alabama

In many countries, the most commonly used vehicle for road transport is a utility bicycle. These have frames with relaxed geometry, protecting the rider from shocks of the road and easing steering at low speeds. Utility bicycles tend to be equipped with accessories such as mudguards, pannier racks and lights, which extends their usefulness on a daily basis. As the bicycle is so effective as a means of transportation various companies have developed methods of carrying anything from the weekly shop to children on bicycles. Certain countries rely heavily on bicycles and their culture has developed around the bicycle as a primary form of transport. In Europe, Denmark and the Netherlands have the most bicycles per capita and most often use bicycles for everyday transport.

Road bikes tend to have a more upright shape and a shorter wheelbase, which make the bike more mobile but harder to ride slowly. The design, coupled with low or dropped handlebars, requires the rider to bend forward more, making use of stronger muscles (particularly the gluteus maximus) and reducing air resistance at high speed.

The price of a new bicycle can range from US$50 to more than US$20,000 (the highest priced bike in the world is the custom Madone by Damien Hirst, sold at $500,000 USD), depending on quality, type and weight (the most exotic road bicycles can weigh as little as 3.2 kg (7 lb)). However, UCI regulations stipulate a legal race bike cannot weigh less than 6.8 kg (14.99 lbs). Being measured for a bike and taking it for a test ride are recommended before buying.

The drivetrain components of the bike should also be considered. A middle grade dérailleur is sufficient for a beginner, although many utility bikes are equipped with hub gears. If the rider plans a significant amount of hillclimbing a triple-chainrings crankset gear system may be preferred. Otherwise, the relatively lighter and less expensive double chainring may be better. Much simpler fixed wheel bikes are also available.

Many road bikes, along with mountain bikes, include clipless pedals to which special shoes attach, via a cleat, enabling the rider to pull on the pedals as well as push. Other possible accessories for the bicycle include front and rear lights, bells or horns, child carrying seats, cycling computers with GPS, locks, bar tape, fenders (mud-guards), baggage racks, baggage carriers and pannier bags, water bottles and bottle cages.

For basic maintenance and repairs cyclists can carry a pump (or a CO_2 cartridge), a puncture repair kit, a spare inner tube, and tire levers and a set of allen keys. Cycling can be more efficient and comfortable with special shoes, gloves, and shorts. In wet weather, riding can be more tolerable with waterproof clothes, such as cape, jacket, trousers (pants) and overshoes and high-visibility clothing is advisable to reduce the risk from motor vehicle users.

Items legally required in some jurisdictions, or voluntarily adopted for safety reasons, include bicycle helmets, generator or battery operated lights, reflectors, and audible signalling devices such as a bell or horn. Extras include studded tires and a bicycle computer.

Bikes can also be heavily customized, with different seat designs and handle bars, for example.

Skills

Many schools and police departments run educational programs to instruct children in bicycle handling skills and introduce them to the rules of the road as they apply to cyclists. In different countries these may be known as bicycle rodeos or operated as schemes such as Bikeability. Education for adult cyclists is available from organizations such as the League of American Bicyclists.

Beyond simply riding, another skill is riding efficiently and safely in traffic. One popular approach to riding in motor vehicle traffic is vehicular cycling, occupying road space as car does. Alternately, in countries such as Denmark and the Netherlands, where cycling is popular, cyclists are often segregated into bike lanes at the side of, or more often separate from, main highways and roads. Many primary schools participate in the national road test in which children individually complete a circuit on roads near the school while being observed by testers.

Infrastructure

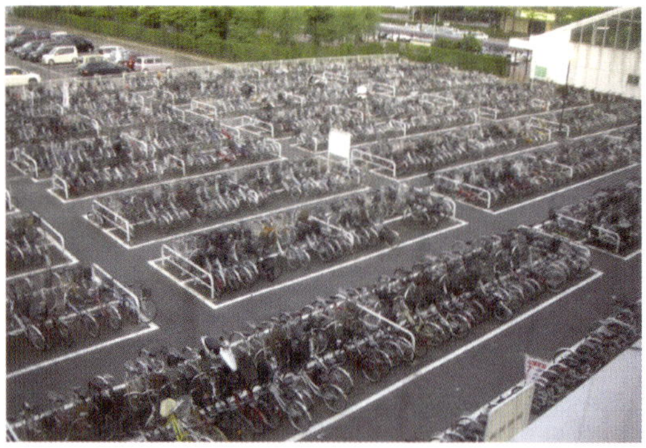

A parking lot for bicycles in Niigata, Japan.

Cyclists, pedestrians and motorists make different demands on road design which may lead to conflicts. Some jurisdictions give priority to motorized traffic, for example setting up one-way street systems, free-right turns, high capacity roundabouts, and slip roads. Others share priority with cyclists so as to encourage more cycling by applying varying combinations of traffic calming measures to limit the impact of motorized transport, and by building bike lanes, bike paths and cycle tracks.

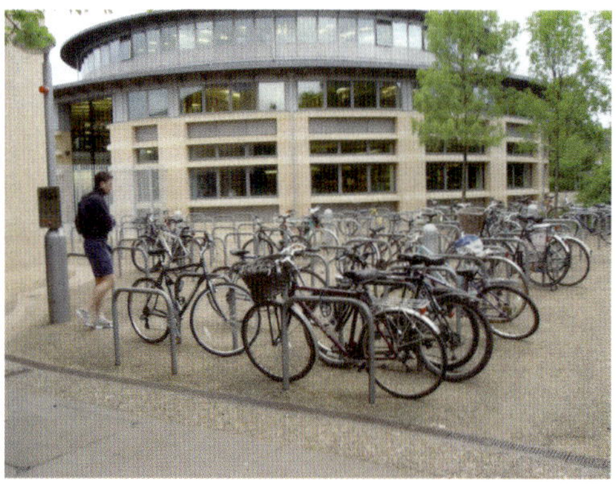

Bicycle stands outside the Centre for Mathematical Sciences at the University of Cambridge. Many students at the university opt to travel by bicycle.

In jurisdictions where motor vehicles were given priority, cycling has tended to decline while in jurisdictions where cycling infrastructure was built, cycling rates have remained steady or increased. Occasionally, extreme measures against cycling may occur. In Shanghai, where bicycles were once the dominant mode of transport, bicycle travel on a few city roads was banned temporarily in December 2003.

In areas in which cycling is popular and encouraged, cycle-parking facilities using bicycle stands, lockable mini-garages, and patrolled cycle parks are used in order to reduce theft. Local governments promote cycling by permitting bicycles to be carried on public transport or by providing external attachment devices on public transport vehicles. Conversely, an absence of secure cycle-parking is a recurring complaint by cyclists from cities with low modal share of cycling.

Extensive cycling infrastructure may be found in some cities. Such dedicated paths in some cities often have to be shared with in-line skaters, scooters, skateboarders, and pedestrians. Dedicated cycling infrastructure is treated differently in the law of every jurisdiction, including the question of liability of users in a collision. There is also some debate about the safety of the various types of separated facilities.

Bicycles are considered a sustainable mode of transport, especially suited for urban use and relatively shorter distances when used for transport (compared to recreation). Case studies and good practices (from European cities and some worldwide examples) that promote and stimulate this kind of functional cycling in cities can be found at Eltis, Europe's portal for local transport.

A number of cities, including Paris, London and Barcelona, now have successful bike hire schemes designed to help people cycle in the city. Typically these feature utilitarian city bikes which lock into docking stations, released on payment for set time periods. Costs vary from city to city. In London, initial hire access costs £2 per day. The first 30 minutes of each trip is free, with £2 for each additional 30 minutes until the bicycle is returned.

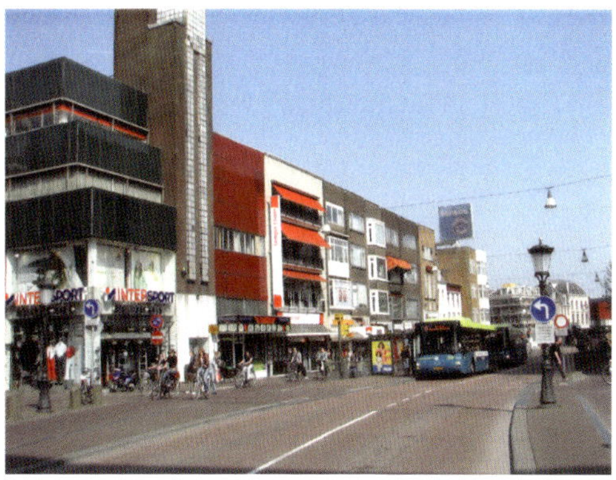

The safe physically separated *Fietspad* in the Netherlands, keeping cyclists away from traffic as seen in Utrecht.

In the Netherlands, many roads have one or two separate cycleways alongside them, or cycle lanes marked on the road. On roads where adjacent bike paths or cycle tracks exist, the use of these facilities is compulsory, and cycling on the main carriageway is not permitted. Some 35,000 km of cycle-track has been physically segregated from motor traffic, equal to a quarter of the country's entire 140,000 km road network.

Types

Utility

Utility cycling refers both to cycling as a mode of daily commuting transport as well as the use of a bicycle in a commercial activity, mainly to transport goods, mostly accomplished in an urban environment.

The postal services of many countries have long relied on bicycles. The British Royal Mail first started using bicycles in 1880; now bicycle delivery fleets include 37,000 in the UK, 25,700 in Germany, 10,500 in Hungary and 7000 in Sweden. In Australia, Australia Post has also reintroduced bicycle postal deliveries on some routes due to an inability to recruit sufficient licensed riders willing to use their uncomfortable motorbikes. The London Ambulance Service has recently introduced bicycling paramedics, who can often get to the scene of an incident in Central London more quickly than a motorized ambulance.

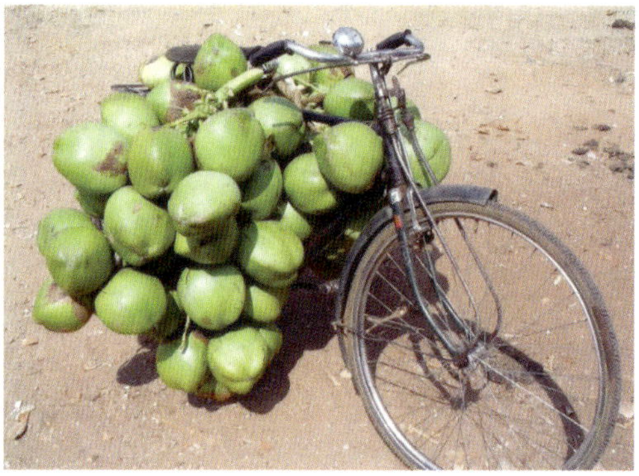

A bicycle loaded with tender coconuts for sale. Karnataka, India.

The use of bicycles by police has been increasing, since they provide greater accessibility to bicycle and pedestrian zones and allow access when roads are congested.

Bicycles enjoy substantial use as general delivery vehicles in many countries. In the UK and North America, as their first jobs, generations of teenagers have worked at delivering newspapers by bicycle. London has many delivery companies that use bicycles with trailers. Most cities in the West, and many outside it, support a sizeable and visible industry of cycle couriers who deliver documents and small packages. In India, many of Mumbai's Dabbawalas use bicycles to deliver home cooked lunches to the city's workers. In Bogotá, Colombia the city's largest bakery recently replaced most of its delivery trucks with bicycles. Even the car industry uses bicycles. At the huge Mercedes-Benz factory in Sindelfingen, Germany workers use bicycles, color-coded by department, to move around the factory.

Recreational

Bicycle Touring

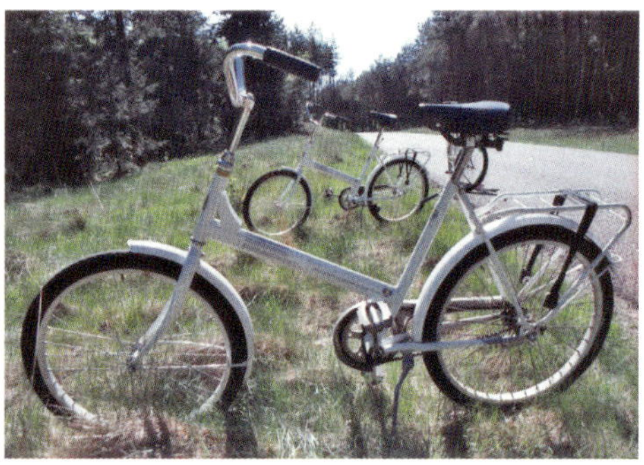

In the Netherlands, bicycles are freely available for use in the Hoge Veluwe National Park.

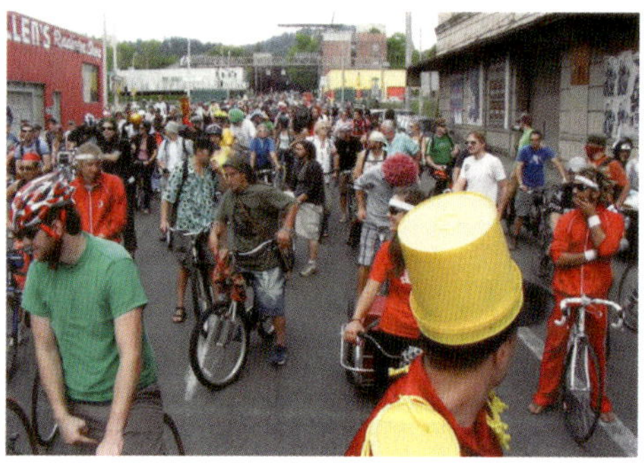

Tour de Fat group ride in Portland, Oregon.

Bicycles are used for recreation at all ages. Bicycle touring, also known as cyclotourism, involves touring and exploration or sightseeing by bicycle for leisure. A brevet or randonnée is an organized long-distance ride.

One popular Dutch pleasure is the enjoyment of relaxed cycling in the countryside of the Netherlands. The land is very flat and full of public bicycle trails and cycle tracks where cyclists are not bothered by cars and other traffic, which makes it ideal for cycling recreation. Many Dutch people subscribe every year to an event called *fietsvierdaagse* — four days of organised cycling through the local environment. Paris–Brest–Paris (PBP), which began in 1891, is the oldest bicycling event still run on a regular basis on the open road, covers over 1,200 km (746 mi) and imposes a 90-hour time limit. Similar if smaller institutions exist in many countries.

Organized Rides

Many cycling clubs hold organized rides in which bicyclists of all levels participate. The typical organized ride starts with a large group of riders, called the mass, bunch or even peloton. This will thin out over the course of the ride. Many riders choose to ride together in groups of the same skill level to take advantage of drafting.

Most organized rides, for example cyclosportives (or gran fondos), Challenge Rides or reliability trials, and hill climbs include registration requirements and will provide information either through the mail or online concerning start times and other requirements. Rides usually consist of several different routes, sorted by mileage, and with a certain number of rest stops that usually include refreshments, first aid and maintenance tools. Routes can vary by as much as 100 miles (160 km).

Mountain

Mountain biking began in the 1970s, originally as a downhill sport, practised on customized cruiser bicycles around Mount Tamalpais. Most mountain biking takes place on dirt roads, trails and in purpose-built parks. Downhill mountain biking has just evolved in the recent years and is performed at places such as Whistler Mountain Bike Park. Slopestyle, a form of downhill, is when riders do tricks such as tailwhips, 360s, backflips and front flips. There are several disciplines of mountain biking besides downhill. Cross country, often referred to as XC, all mountain, trail, free ride, and newly popular enduro.

Other

The Marching and Cycling Band HHK from Haarlem (the Netherlands) is one of the few marching bands around the world which also performs on bicycles.

Racing

Shortly after the introduction of bicycles, competitions developed independently in many parts of the world. Early races involving boneshaker style bicycles were predictably fraught with injuries. Large races became popular during the 1890s "Golden Age of Cycling", with events across Europe, and in the U.S. and Japan as well. At one point, almost every major city in the US had a velodrome or two for track racing events, however since the middle of the 20th century cycling has become a minority sport in the US whilst in Continental Europe it continues to be a major sport, particularly in the United Kingdom, France, Belgium, Italy and Spain. The most famous of all bicycle races is the Tour de France. This began in 1903, and continues to capture the attention of the sporting world.

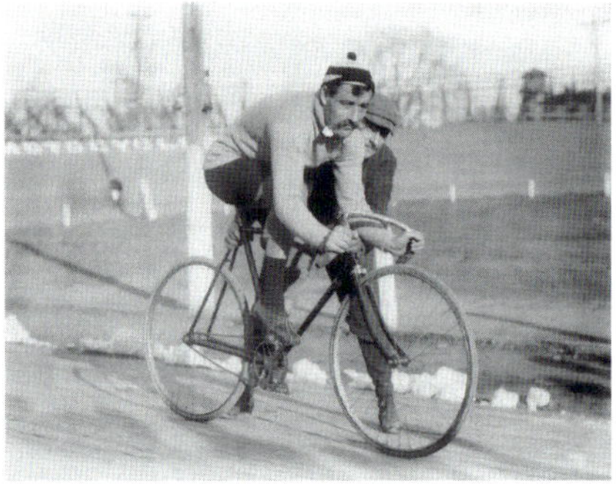

Bicycle racing.

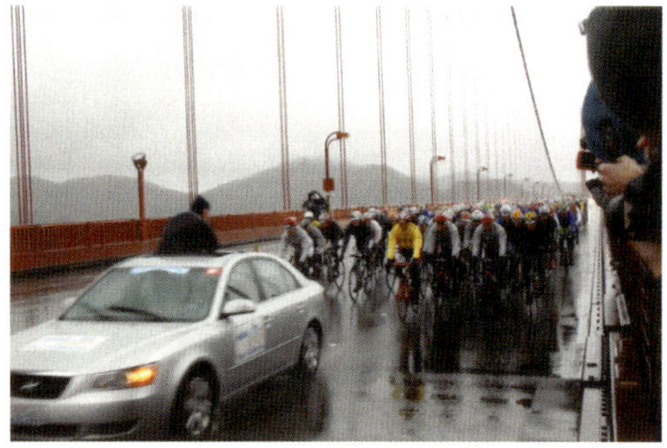

A peloton of professional bicycle racers on the Golden Gate Bridge

In 1899, Charles Minthorn Murphy became the first man to ride his bicycle a mile in under a minute (hence his nickname, Mile-a-Minute Murphy), which he did by drafting a locomotive at New York's Long Island.

As the bicycle evolved its various forms, different racing formats developed. Road races may involve both team and individual competition, and are contested in various ways. They range from the one-day road race, criterium, and time trial to multi-stage events like the Tour de France and its sister events which make up cycling's Grand Tours. Recumbent bicycles were banned from bike races in 1934 after Marcel Berthet set a new hour record in his *Velodyne streamliner* (49.992 km on November 18, 1933). Track bicycles are used for track cycling in Velodromes, while cyclo-cross races are held on outdoor terrain, including pavement, grass, and mud. Cyclocross races feature man-made features such as small barriers which riders either bunny hop over or dismount and walk over. Time trial races, another form of road racing require a rider to ride against the clock. Time trials can be performed as a team or as a single rider. Bikes are changed for time trial races, using aero bars. In the past decade, mountain bike racing has also reached international popularity and is even an Olympic sport.

Professional racing organizations place limitations on the bicycles that can be used in the races that they sanction. For example, the Union Cycliste Internationale, the governing body of international cycle sport (which sanctions races such as the Tour de France), decided in the late 1990s to create additional rules which prohibit racing bicycles weighing less than 6.8 kilograms (14.96 pounds). The UCI rules also effectively ban some bicycle frame innovations (such as the recumbent bicycle) by requiring a double triangle structure.

War

The bicycle has been used as a method of reconnaissance as well as transporting soldiers and supplies to combat zones. In this it has taken over many of the functions of horses in warfare. In the Second Boer War, both sides used bicycles for scouting. In World War I, France, Germany, Australia and New Zealand used bicycles to move troops. In its 1937 invasion of China, Japan employed some 50,000 bicycle troops, and similar forces were instrumental in Japan's march or "roll" through Malaya in World War II. Germany used bicycles again in World War II, while the British employed airborne "Cycle-commandos" with folding bikes.

In the Vietnam War, communist forces used bicycles extensively as cargo carriers along the Ho Chi Minh Trail.

The last country known to maintain a regiment of bicycle troops was Switzerland, which disbanded its last unit in 2003.

Activism

Two broad and correlated themes run in bicycle activism: one is about advocating the bicycle as an alternative mode of transport, and the other is about the creation of conditions to permit and/or encourage bicycle use, both for utility and recreational cycling. Although the first, which emphasizes the potential for energy and resource conservation and health benefits gained from cycling versus automobile use, is relatively undisputed, the second is the subject of much debate.

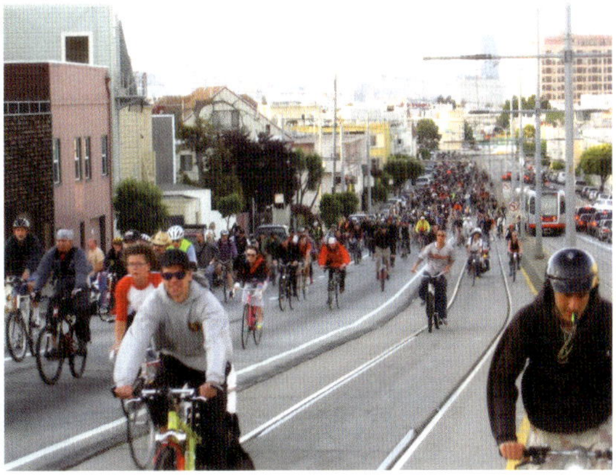

San Francisco Critical Mass.

It is generally agreed that improved local and inter-city rail services and other methods of mass transportation (including greater provision for cycle carriage on such services) create conditions to encourage bicycle use. However, there are different opinions on the role of various types of cycling infrastructure in building bicycle-friendly cities and roads.

Some bicycle activists (including some traffic management advisers) seek the construction of bike paths, cycle tracks and bike lanes for journeys of all lengths and point to their success in promoting safety and encouraging more people to cycle. Some activists, especially those from the vehicular cycling tradition, view the safety, practicality, and intent of such facilities with suspicion. They favor a more holistic approach based on the 4 'E's; *education* (of everyone involved), *encouragement* (to apply the education), *enforcement* (to protect the rights of others), and *engineering* (to facilitate travel while respecting every person's equal right to do so). Some groups offer training courses to help cyclists integrate themselves with other traffic.

Critical Mass is an event typically held on the last Friday of every month in cities around the world where bicyclists take to the streets *en masse*. While the ride was founded with the idea of drawing attention to how unfriendly the city was to bicyclists, the leaderless structure of Critical Mass makes it impossible to assign it any one specific goal. In fact, the purpose of Critical Mass is not formalized beyond the direct action of meeting at a set location and time and traveling as a group through city streets.

There is a long-running cycle helmet debate among activists. The most heated controversy surrounds the topic of compulsory helmet use.

Associations

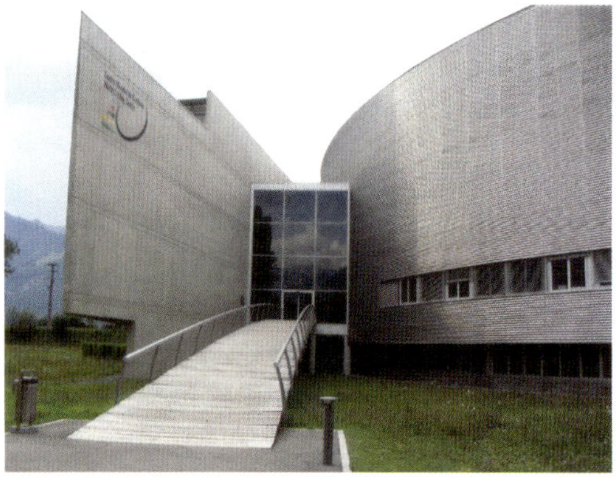

Headquarters of the Union Cycliste Internationale in Switzerland.

Cyclists form associations, both for specific interests (trails development, road maintenance, bike maintenance, urban design, racing clubs, touring clubs, etc.) and for more global goals (energy conservation, pollution reduction, promotion of fitness). Some bicycle clubs and national associations became prominent advocates for improvements to roads and highways. In the United States, the League of American Wheelmen lobbied for the improvement of roads in the last part of the 19th century, founding and leading the national Good Roads Movement. Their model for political organization, as well as the paved roads for which they argued, facilitated the growth of the automobile.

As a sport, cycling is governed internationally by the Union Cycliste Internationale in Switzerland, USA Cycling (merged with the United States Cycling Federation in 1995) in the United States, (for upright bicycles) and by the International Human Powered Vehicle Association (for other HPVs, or human-powered vehicles). Cycling for transport and touring is promoted on a European level by the European Cyclists' Federation, with associated members from Great Britain, Japan and elsewhere. Regular conferences on cycling as transport are held under the auspices of Velo City; global conferences are coordinated by Velo Mondial.

Health effects

The health benefits of cycling outweigh the risks, when cycling is compared to a sedentary lifestyle. A Dutch study found that cycling can extend lifespans by up to 14 months, but the risks equated to a reduced lifespan of 40 days or less. Cycling in the Netherlands is often safer than in other parts of the world, so the risk-benefit ratio will be different in other regions. Overall, benefits of cycling or walking have been shown to exceed risks by ratios of 9:1 to 96:1 when compared with no exercise at all.

Exercise

The physical exercise gained from cycling is generally linked with increased health and well-being. According to the World Health Organization, physical inactivity is second only to tobacco smoking as a health risk in developed countries, and this is associated with many tens of billions of dollars of healthcare costs. The WHO's report suggests that increasing physical activity is a public health 'best buy', and that cycling is a 'highly suitable activity' for this purpose. The charity Sustrans reports that investment in cycling provision can give a 20:1 return from health and other benefits. It has been estimated that, on average, approximately 20 life-years are gained from the health benefits of road bicycling for every life-year lost through injury.

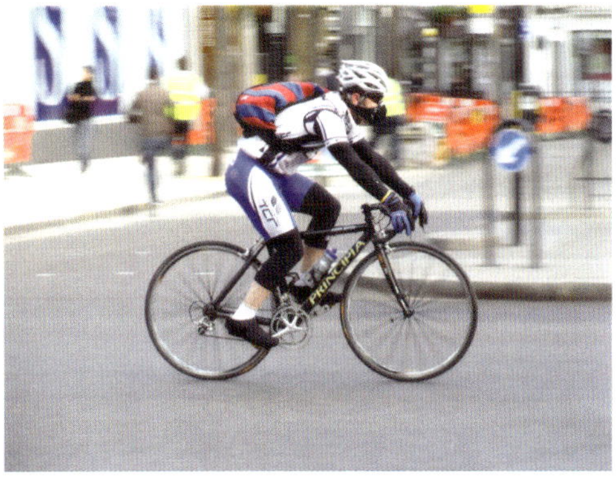

Heavily equipped London cyclist: specialist cycle clothing, pollution mask, dark glasses and helmet.

Bicycles are often used by people seeking to improve their fitness and cardiovascular health. In this regard, cycling is especially helpful for those with arthritis of the lower limbs who are unable to pursue sports that cause impact to the knees and other joints. Since cycling can be used for the practical purpose of transportation, there can be less need for self-discipline to exercise.

Cycling while seated is a relatively non-weight bearing exercise that, like swimming, does little to promote bone density. Cycling up and out of the saddle, on the other hand, does a better job by transferring more of the rider's body weight to the legs. However, excessive cycling while standing can cause knee damage It used to be thought that cycling while standing was less energy efficient, but recent research has proven this not to be true. Other than air resistance, there is no wasted energy from cycling while standing, if it is done correctly.

Cycling on a stationary cycle is frequently advocated as a suitable exercise for rehabilitation, particularly for lower limb injury, owing to the low impact which it has on the joints. In particular, cycling is commonly used within knee rehabilitation programs.

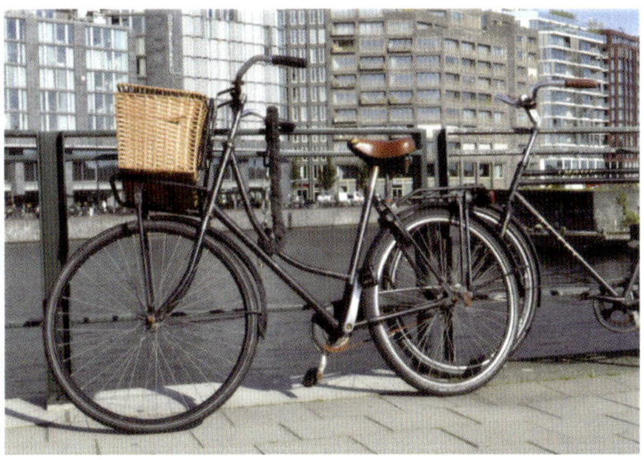

Bike at Prins Hendrikkade Amsterdam.

As a response to the increased global sedentarity and consequent overweight and obesity, one response that has been adopted by many organizations concerned with health and environment is the promotion of Active travel, which seeks to promote walking and cycling as safe and attractive alternatives to motorized transport. Given that many journeys are for relatively short distances, there is considerable scope to replace car use with walking or cycling, though in many settings this may require some infrastructure modification, particularly to attract the less experienced and confident.

Bicycle Safety

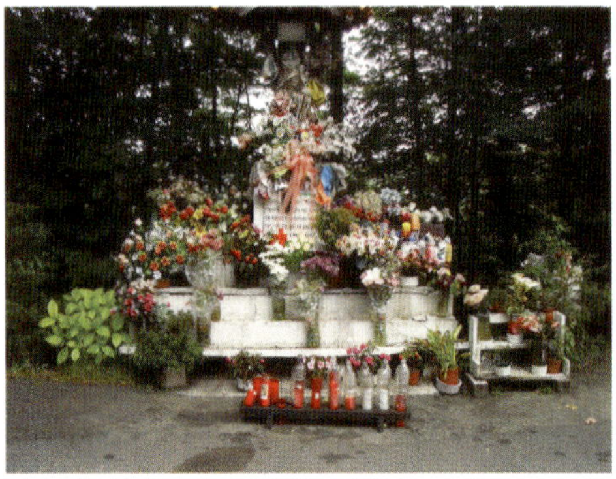

Virgin Mary venerated as the holy protector of bicyclists on the roads of the mountainous Basque Country.

Cycling suffers from a perception that it is unsafe. This perception is not always backed by hard numbers, because of under reporting of accidents and lack of bicycle use data (amount of cycling, kilometers cycled) which make it hard to assess the risk and monitor changes in risks.In the UK, fatality rates per mile or kilometre are slightly less than those for walking. In the US, bicycling fatality rates are less than 2/3 of those walking the same distance. However, in the UK for example the fatality and serious injury rates *per hour of travel* are just over double for cycling than those for walking. Thus if a person is, for example, about to undertake a ten kilometre journey to a given destination it may on average be safer to undertake this journey by bicycle than on foot. However, if a person is intending, for example, to undertake an hour's exercise it may be more dangerous to take that exercise by cycling rather than by walking.

Despite the risk factors associated with bicycling, cyclists have a lower overall mortality rate when compared to other groups. A Danish study in 2000 found that even after adjustment for other risk factors, including leisure time physical activity, those who did not cycle to work experienced a 39% higher mortality rate than those who did.

Injuries (to cyclists, from cycling) can be divided into two types:

- Physical trauma (extrinsic)
- Overuse (intrinsic).

Physical Trauma

Acute physical trauma includes injuries to the head and extremities resulting from falls and collisions. Most cycle deaths result from a collision with a car or heavy goods vehicle, both motorist and cyclist having been found responsible for collisions. A third of collisions between motorists and cyclists are caused by car dooring. However, around 16% of serious cyclist injuries reported to police in the UK in 2014 did not involve any other person or vehicle.

Although a majority of bicycle collisions occur during the day, bicycle lighting is recommended for safety when bicycling at night to increase visibility.

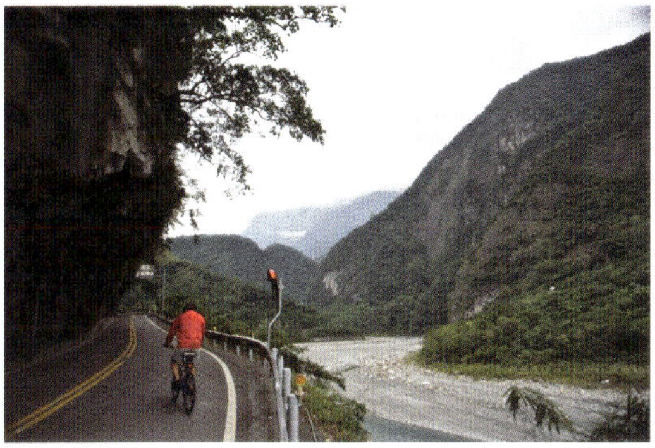

Bicyclist pedals uphill at the Taroko Gorge in Taiwan.

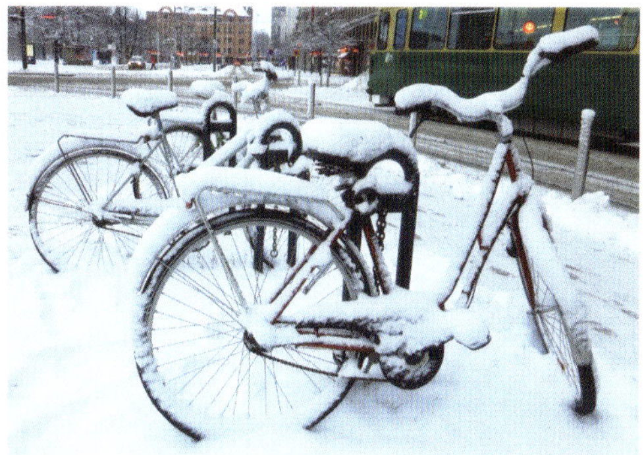

Bicycles in Helsinki (Finland).

Overuse Injuries

Of a study of 518 cyclists, a large majority reported at least one overuse injury, with over one third requiring medical treatment. The most common injury sites were the neck (48.8%) and the knees (41.7%), as well as the groin/buttocks (36.1%), hands (31.1%), and back (30.3%). Women were more likely to suffer from neck and shoulder pain than men.

Many cyclists suffer from overuse injuries to the knees, affecting cyclists at all levels. These are caused by many factors:

- Incorrect bicycle fit or adjustment, particularly the saddle.
- Incorrect adjustment of clipless pedals.
- Too many hills, or too many miles, too early in the training season.
- Poor training preparation for long touring rides.
- Selecting too high a gear. A lower gear for uphill climb protects the knees, even though muscles may be well able to handle a higher gear.

Overuse injuries, including chronic nerve damage at weight bearing locations, can occur as a result of repeatedly riding a bicycle for extended periods of time. Damage to the ulnar nerve in the palm, carpal tunnel in the wrist, the genitourinary tract or bicycle seat neuropathy may result from overuse. Recumbent bicycles are designed on different ergonomic principles and eliminate pressure from the saddle and handlebars, due to the relaxed riding position.

Note that overuse is a relative term, and capacity varies greatly between individuals. Someone starting out in cycling must be careful to increase length and frequency of cycling sessions slowly, starting for example at an hour or two per day, or a hundred miles or kilometers per week. Bilateral muscular pain is a normal by-product of the training process, whereas unilateral pain may reveal "exercise-induced arterial endofibrosis". Joint pain and numbness are also early signs of overuse injury.

A Spanish study of top triathletes found those who cover more than 186 miles (300 km) a week on their bikes have less than 4% normal looking sperm, where normal adult males would be expected to have from 15% to 20%.

Saddle Related

Much work has been done to investigate optimal bicycle saddle shape, size and position, and negative effects of extended use of less than optimal seats or configurations.

Excessive saddle height can cause posterior knee pain, while setting the saddle too low can cause pain in the anterior of the knee. An incorrectly fitted saddle may eventually lead to muscle imbalance. A 25 to 35 degree knee angle is recommended to avoid an overuse injury.

Cycling has been linked to sexual impotence due to pressure on the perineum from the seat, but fitting a proper sized seat prevents this effect. In extreme cases, pudendal nerve entrapment can be a source of intractable perineal pain. Some cyclists with induced pudendal nerve pressure neuropathy gained relief from improvements in saddle position and riding techniques.

The National Institute for Occupational Safety and Health (NIOSH) has investigated the potential health effects of prolonged bicycling in police bicycle patrol units, including the possibility that some bicycle saddles exert excessive pressure on the urogenital area of cyclists, restricting blood flow to the genitals. Their study found that using bicycle seats without protruding noses reduced pressure on the groin by at least 65% and significantly reduced the number of cases of urogenital paresthesia. A follow-up found that 90% of bicycle officers who tried the no-nose seat were using it six months later. NIOSH recommends that riders use a no-nose bicycle seat for workplace bicycling.

Despite rumors to the contrary, there is no scientific evidence linking cycling with testicular cancer.

Exposure to Air Pollution

One concern is that riding in traffic may expose the cyclist to higher levels of air pollution, especially if he or she travels on or along busy roads. Some authors have claimed this to be untrue, showing that the pollutant and irritant count within cars is consistently higher, presumably because of limited circulation of air within the car and due to the air intake being directly in the stream of other traffic. Other authors have found small or inconsistent differences in concentrations but claim that exposure of cyclists is higher due to increased minute ventilation and is associated with minor biological changes. The significance of the associated health effect, if any, is unclear but probably much smaller than the health impacts associated with accidents and the health benefits derived from additional physical activity.

Outdoor Rowing

Rowing as a sport was initiated on the River Thames. Professional watermen competed in the Doggett Coat and Badge Race. "Gentlemen" began competing in 1829 with the Oxford-Cambridge race. The Henly Regatta was started in 1839. Competitve rowing crossed the Atlantic and the Yale-Harvard race was introduced n the Charles river in 1852. Rowing was the first organized collegiate sport in the United States, complete with its own governing body. Today, collegiate rowing in the U.S. remains independent of the NCAA. International championships were first arranged in 1893, and remain under the direction of the Federation International des Societes d' Aviron (FISA).

Attributes Needed for Rowing

Generally youths start to row at around 13 years of age. There are no special physical attributes necessary except the willingness to learn and have a positive attitude. The youths should also be able to swim as it is nearly certain that at some stage they will fall from the boat while learning to row. Coxing is also a very important activity that does not require any fitness level. Coxing can also suit a person who may not be able to row but might want to experience the comradeship of participation. If fact you can start to row at any age and is not restricted to youths. There is a novice and masters scene also.

Types of Rowing

Sweep and scull. Sweep rowing involves one long oar, held with both hands. The minimum in a boat is two, one person rowing on each side.

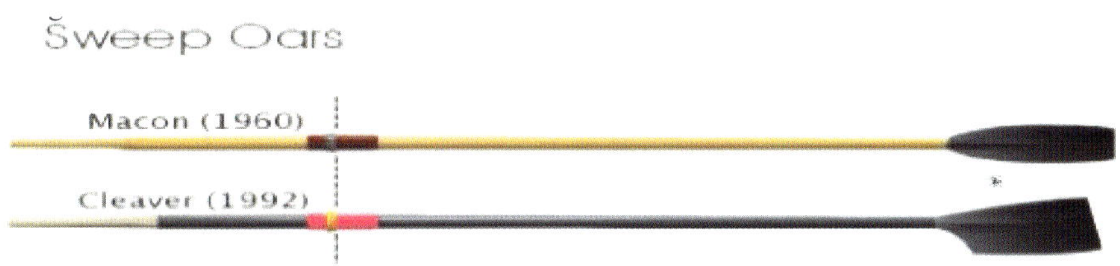

In sculling boats, each rower has two smaller oars, one in each hand. Although, sculling can be done in multi-person boats, it is the only style that can be done individually.

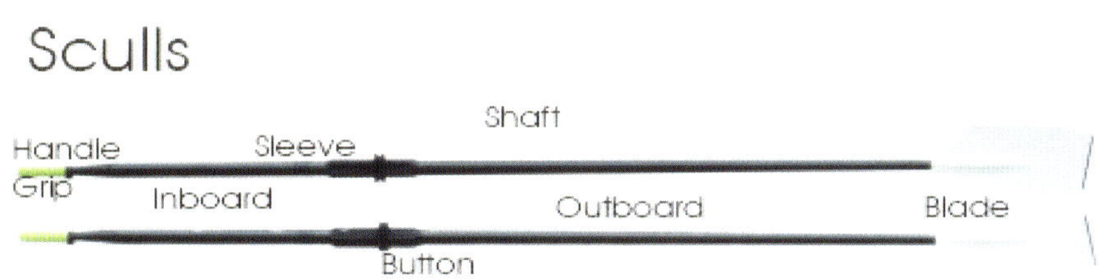

Both rowing styles are fun. Sweep rowing has a tendency to develop one side of the body. Sculling allows a more uniform development and is what all new members will be taught first. More emphasis is put on sculling for all junior rowers.

Boats

The below table shows all the possible boat types. A few types are expanded upon for you the reader to understand the terminology better.

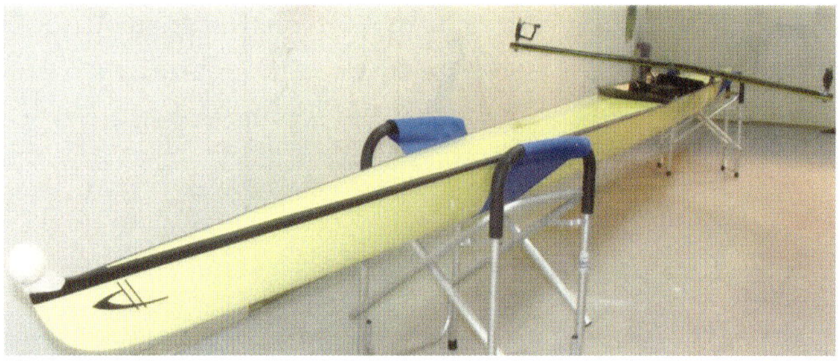

- Single (1X) One rower or sculler. Singles are about 8m long and less than 0.3m wide. Racing singles can weigh as little as 13.5kg.
- Coxed Pair (2+) Two sweep rowers with a coxswain.
- Coxless Pair (2-) Two sweep rowers without a coxswain.
- Coxed Four (4+) Four sweep rowers with a coxswain.
- Coxless Four (4) Four sweep rowers without a coxswain.

Steering is usually accomplished via a rudder that is attached to a cable that is connected to one of the rower's foot stretchers (this an adjustable bracket to which the rower's feet are secured). The coxless pair has a similar type of rudder setup.

- Eight(8+/8o) Eight sweep rowers with a coxswain. Eights are(~18.5m) long and weigh about (114kg).

Number of People	Name	Symbol		Name	Symbol
8	Eight	VIII+,8+		Octuple	8x+
4	Coxed four	IV+, 4+		Coxed quad	4x+
4	Coxless four	IV-, 4-		Coxless quad	4x-
2	Coxed pair	2+		-	-
2	Coxless pair	2-		Double	2x-
1	Single	1x-		-	-

Note:
+ means there is a cox.
– means there is no cox.
x *means its a scull i.e. the person has two oars.*

Training for Rowing

Rowing training is broken down into land-based and water-based training.

Land-based Training:

- Running.
- Ergometer (a rowing machine that monitors the rower's performance – often referred to as an erg).
- Circuit training i.e. push ups, sit ups and general body exercises.

- Resistance training with weights. (Generally restricted until oars people are over 15 years of age.)

Water-based Training:

- Technical drills in the rowing boat.
- Season-specific fitness training.

References

- Rodriguez, Robert G. (2009). The Regulation of Boxing: A History and Comparative Analysis of Policies Among American States. McFarland. ISBN 9780786438624.
- Genin, J. J. Willems, P. A.; Cavagna, G. A.; Lair, R.; Heglund, N. C. (2010). "Biomechanics of locomotion in Asian elephants". Journal of Experimental Biology. 213 (5): 694–706. doi:10.1242/jeb.035436. PMID 20154184.
- SA, WebSide Associates. "The Official World Rowing Web Site - Rowing / Ergometer/Indoor". wayback.archive.org. Archived from the original on 10 November 2006. Retrieved 15 May 2017.
- Church TS, Earnest CP, Morss GM (2013-03-25). "Field testing of physiological responses associated with Nordic Walking". Res Q Exerc Sport. 73: 296–300. doi:10.1080/02701367.2002.10609023. PMID 12230336.
- Tolley, Rodney (2003). Sustainable transport: planning for walking and cycling in urban environments. Woodhead Publishing. p. 72. ISBN 1-85573-614-4.
- Hutchinson, J. R.; Schwerda, D.; Famini, D. J.; Dale, R. H.; Fischer, M. S. Kram, R. (2006). "The locomotor kinematics of Asian and African elephants: changes with speed and size". Journal of Experimental Biology. 209 (19): 3812–27. doi:10.1242/jeb.02443. PMID 16985198.
- "Relationship of walking to mortality among U.S. adults". Centers for Disease Control. 20 May 2011. Archived from the original on 29 January 2013. Retrieved 16 October 2013.
- H. Jung et al. The ancient origins of neural substrates for land walking. Cell. Vol. 172, February 8, 2018, p. 667. doi: 10.1016/j.cell.2018.01.013

Chapter 4

Swimming: Water Exercise

Swimming is a recreational activity, an exercise or a sport involved with the self-propulsion of an individual in water using his/her arms and legs. The aim of this chapter is to explore the principal topics of resistance swimming and swimming stroke with respect to physical education. It explores the different types of swimming strokes, such as front crawl, butterfly stroke, breaststroke, backstroke, sidestroke, etc.

Swimming, in recreation and sports, the propulsion of the body through water by combined arm and leg motions and the natural flotation of the body. Swimming as an exercise is popular as an all-around body developer and is particularly useful in therapy and as exercise for physically handicapped persons. It is also taught for lifesaving purposes.

Instruction and Training

The earliest instruction programs were in Great Britain in the 19th century, both for sport and for lifesaving. Those programs were copied in the rest of Europe. In the United States swimming instruction for lifesaving purposes began under the auspices of the American Red Cross in 1916. Instructional work done by the various branches of the armed forces during both World Wars I and II was very effective in promoting swimming. Courses taught by community organizations and schools, extending ultimately to very young infants, became common.

The early practice of simply swimming as much as possible at every workout was replaced by interval training and repeat training by the late 1950s. Interval training consists of a series of swims of the same distance with controlled rest periods. In slow interval training, used primarily to develop endurance, the rest period is always shorter than the time taken to swim the prescribed distance. Fast interval training, used primarily to develop speed, permits rest periods long enough to allow almost complete recovery of the heart and breathing rate.

The increased emphasis on international competition led to the growing availability of 50-metre (164-foot) pools. Other adjuncts that improved both training and performance included wave-killing gutters for pools, racing lane markers that also reduce turbulence, cameras for underwater study of strokes, large clocks visible to swimmers, and electrically operated touch and timing devices. Since 1972 all world records have been expressed in hundredths of a second. Advances in swimsuit technology reached a head at the 2008 Olympic Games in Beijing, where swimmers—wearing high-tech bodysuits that increased buoyancy and decreased water resistance—broke 25 world records. After another round of record-shattering times at the 2009 world championships, FINA banned such bodysuits, for fear that they augmented a competitor's true ability.

Health Benefits of Swimming

Swimming is a great workout because you need to move your whole body against the resistance of the water.

Swimming is a good all-round activity because it:

- keeps your heart rate up but takes some of the impact stress off your body
- builds endurance, muscle strength and cardiovascular fitness
- helps maintain a healthy weight, healthy heart and lungs
- tones muscles and builds strength
- provides an all-over body workout, as nearly all of your muscles are used during swimming.

Other Benefits of Swimming

Swimming has many other benefits including:

- being a relaxing and peaceful form of exercise
- alleviating stress
- improving coordination, balance and posture
- improving flexibility
- providing good low-impact therapy for some injuries and conditions
- providing a pleasant way to cool down on a hot day

Resistance Swimming

Resistance training is, as the name implies, getting your muscles to contract against an external form of resistance, such as dumbbells, exercise bands, your own body weight, a block of cement, soup cans or any other external object. Resistance training is good for your overall level of fitness because it increases your strength, muscle tone, muscle mass and your endurance. There are three types of resistance training including Olympic lifting, powerlifting and weightlifting, but swimming is not included in the group of resistance exercises.

If you are still confused as to why exerting yourself against a body of water does not constitute resistance training, you need to examine further how resistance training actually works. As harsh as it sounds, resistance training works because you actually tear your muscles while exerting against a weight. In your off-workout periods, your body repairs these tears, making itself stronger. Even though moving through water offers more resistance than moving through air, water does not exert sufficient force on your muscles to tear them, so it is not classified as a resistance exercise.

Although gliding through the water does not provide sufficient resistance to get you the muscles of a female bodybuilder, swimming allows you to tone your body without applying a harsh impact to your skeleton, which is typical of other aerobic exercises and resistance training moves. The resistance offered by swimming is 12 times as dense as air, according to the Discovery Fit & Health website. So jumping into the pool may be a good way to get your body used to adding some resistance without pumping iron.

Tethered Swimming

In its most simple form, it consists of swimming while being held relatively stationary by a flexible restraining device, such as a harness or a foot restraint. This training method is used by a number of swim teams, such as the ones at Purdue University, University of Indianapolis, Florida State University and the University of Florida. Likewise, Special Forces Scuba Team members at Fort Bragg use a commercial restraining device in their personal training for open water swimming. Users often indicate that it takes a certain amount of time to learn to compensate for the feeling of swimming against a restraint. However, for those who have familiarized themselves with these systems, tethers enable the swimmer to swim at any speed, even flat-out sprints, and to vary the speed at will.

Tethered swimming, as this method is known, has been in use since the middle of the twentieth century, and has undergone a gradual evolution. Initially the swimmers were restrained by a rope, which was eventually supplanted by interlocked bicycle inner tubes or surgical tubing. Presently the systems in use employ either bungee cords or coiled lines to provide the shock-absorption necessary for a comfortable swim. Attachment methods also vary. Some devices restrain the swimmer by means of a belt, others wrap around the ankles, and still others connect to specially modified water shoes.

Hybrid Systems

These swimming machines straddle the difference between traditional tethers and mechanical swimming machines. As a result, they combine the advantages of both, with a couple of drawbacks. They share the self-contained aspect of counter-current swimming machines with the low cost, simplicity and freedom of movement of tether systems. They are not strictly speaking "still-water pools" since the movements of the swimmer actually induce a gentle current of water which permits a more natural swimming experience. There are no energy costs (other than the water quality system) with these machines, as they use no electricity for swimming. While they are valuable for aerobic exercise, endurance and strength training, and for stroke practice, they cannot replicate open water conditions. Thus, for competition training they have to be complemented with open-water practice.

Swimming Machines

Another form of resistance swimming is that in which the swimmer is unrestrained and the water is set in motion by means of mechanical devices, such as jets, propellers or paddle wheels. Such an apparatus is also known as a *countercurrent swimming machine*, of which a number are presently available commercially. A prototype machine was used by the Columbia University swim team in the late 1980s.

Swimming machines made their appearance in the 1970s, initially in the form of jetted streams. Some of these were criticized for causing turbulence and an un-natural swimming environment. They were followed by paddle-wheel and propeller-driven machines, which were popularized by Endless Pools. These generated a smoother stream of water. Many users find them easy to swim in, but the machines are also criticized for being expensive, noisy, and wasteful of energy (consuming 6.5 kW to 11 kW of electricity just to set the water in motion).

Finally, there are exercise machines which allow a person to remain on dry land while simulating certain swimming strokes. These devices however can not compensate for the weight of the body and the limbs and thus deprive the user of the benefits of exercise in an aquatic environment.

Tools used to Create the Resistance

1. Stretch cords, you can now make swimming against resistance much more a central part of your workout regime. What's more, it's not going to cost you an arm and a leg to do so. Stretch cords are easy and cheap to get hold of. Yet, they can offer a huge difference to the effectiveness of your workout. It is often true that the simplest items can make the biggest difference to your workout, and this is just yet another example of that being the case. Simply attach one end of the stretch cord to your waist, and the other either to an anchor or ask a friend to hold it, you then simply swim out as fast and as powerfully as you can. The benefit of stretch cords is they provide the highest possible level of resistance.

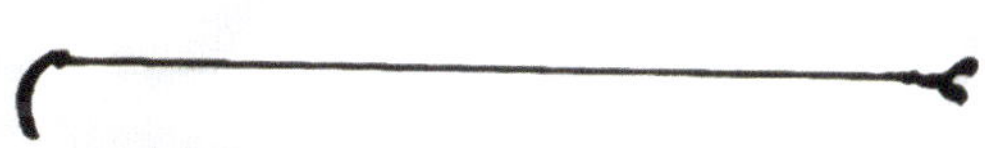

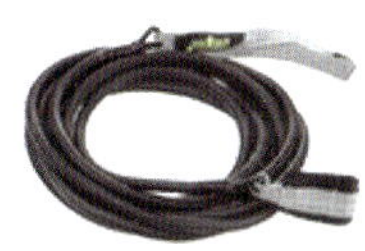

2. Drag tights & shorts, unisex drag tights look and feel great, they provide additional drag while swimming and are a great tool for swimming in public pool. Drag tights and shorts offer the benefit of being able to move freely in a pool, meaning they can be used during public sessions and you won't be getting in the way. You may find that due to the loose nature of drag shorts, they provide more drag than tights, both are unisex and designed to be worn under/over your normal swimwear.

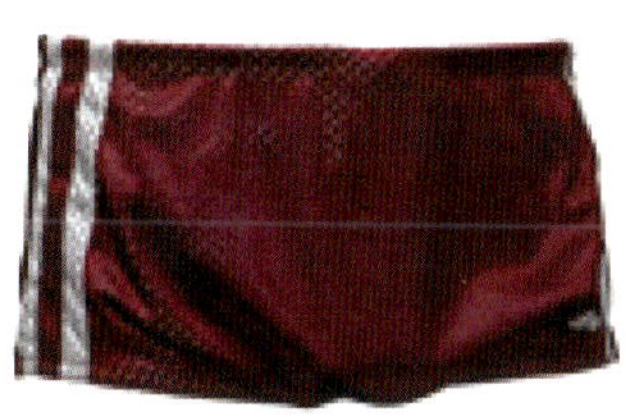

3. Drag Belt, drag belts combine heavy resistance while still allowing you to be mobile in the water. Featuring cups around the edge, the belt can provide an excellent level of resistance

at a low cost. Designed to increase both strength and stamina, yet still fit easily in your gear bag!

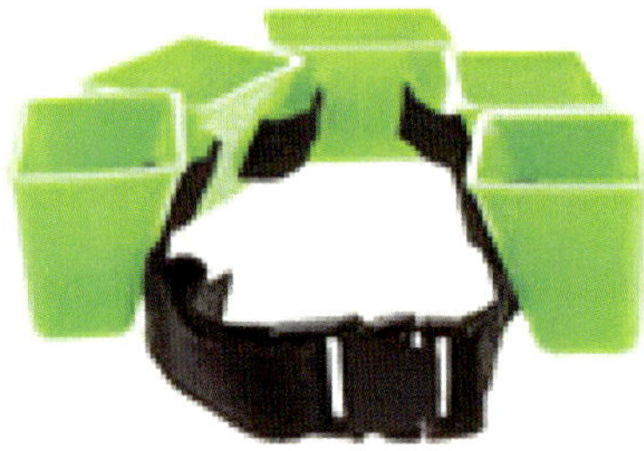

Safety

Why would you want to use resistance in your swimming training sessions? Well, it turns out that using resistance in the water can be a powerful way to make your workouts more effective. Plus, it's not just swimmers who might use the water to work out. Athletes of all kinds can find huge benefits from resistance training in the water.

For a start, resistance training reduces the stress on your joints and muscles, due to the buoyant nature of the water itself. You can also expect to achieve the desired level of muscle tone considerably faster. And something that a lot of people finds useful: you will almost always burn more calories working out in this way, as it will take more muscle energy to push through the water - especially with the added resistance of the stretch cords.

Stretch cords easily provide the most resistance, drag shorts & tights probably look the best, and belts are the most convenient. All of the resistance accessories will certainly help build your strength and stamina, it's just a case of choosing the right one for you! If you want to build your stroke strength or your swimming technique, they might prove to be the essential item. Please be wary the first time you use resistance training accessories as it is common people under estimate the resistance they provide and occasionally get left stranded in the middle of the pool an-able to go much further.

Swimming Stroke

A method of moving the arms and legs to push against the water and propel the swimmer forward is called swimming stroke.

Basic Strokes of Swimming

Dog Paddle

Often the first stroke a young swimmer learns, the dog paddle is very basic, easy to learn and allows you to keep your head above the water for easy breathing. The stroke mimics the movements of a four-legged animal as you propel through the water. You extend your arms forward and your hands alternate as they paw at the water moving in a downward, circular movement. Your legs extend backward with bent knees and your feet alternate in a quick up and down movement to perform a flutter kick.

Backstroke

Sometimes referred to as a back crawl, the backstroke is the fastest stroke performed on your back. Your arms alternate the pushing and pulling parts of the stroke with a circular, windmill motion. As one arm extends forward and enters the water, the other is exiting. Your legs alternate in an up-and-down motion, to perform the flutter kick. Your face is out of the water, which allows you to develop your own breathing pattern.

Freestyle

Sometimes referred to as the crawl, the freestyle is one of the fastest strokes. It is performed on your stomach with your face in the water and your whole body close to the surface. Similar to the backstroke, your arms move in a circular, windmill motion and you use the flutter kick. Your arms alternate, as one arm reaches forward, enters and starts to pull through the water, the other arm exists the water. To breathe, instead of lifting your head, turn it to one side to take a quick breath.

Sidestroke

The sidestroke is performed while on your right or left side. The stroke starts with your bottom arm extending forward, above your head, your palm down and your top arm resting along your side. Simultaneously, pull your bottom arm backward in a sweeping, half-circular motion to the front of your chest, bend your top arm slightly and move it forward to the front of your chest. Your top arm then sweeps backward until it is fully extended. After a short glide you repeat the arm movements. The sidestroke uses a scissor kick -- you move your legs back and forth the way scissors open and close.

Breaststroke

The breaststroke is more complex, requires precise timing and is performed on your stomach with your face in the water. Your arms extend forward, below the water, pull backward in an outward sweeping motion toward your chest and then extend again to glide and start the next stroke. As you pull your arms back, you lift your head to breathe. The frog kick is used and starts when your arms begin to reach forward to glide. You bend your knees, bring your feet up toward your body, move your feet outward and then extend and snap your legs together.

Butterfly

The butterfly stroke also requires precise timing in addition to coordination. You time the movement of your arms with a dolphin kick as your body undulates, similar to the way worms move, through the water. Lift both arms out of the water, reach forward, enter the water in front of your shoulders and pull your hands back through the water toward your feet. When your hands are near your thighs, lift your head to breathe, lift your arms out of the water and repeat the stroke. Take two dolphin kicks with each stroke. Keep your legs together, bend your knees and whip your feet downward.

Special Purpose Styles

A number of strokes are only used for special purposes, e.g. to manipulate an object (a swimmer in distress, a ball), or just to stay afloat.

Underwater Swimming

Any style with underwater recovery can be done underwater for certain distances depending on the need for air. Underwater swimming on the back has the additional problem of water entering the nose. To avoid this, the swimmer can breathe out through the nose or wear a nose clip. Some swimmers can close their nostrils with the upper lip or with the compressor naris muscles.

- Pull-down Breaststroke: most common swim stroke underwater as it requests very low energy. Main application is for dynamic apnea (DNF)
- Dolphin kick: really fast underwater swimming style e.g. Ryan Lochte 50m Underwater - 20.8 SCY
- Sea lion stroke: this swimming stroke is primarily performed with sculling, arms at the side along the bodyline and strongly supported with flutter kicks in a contralateral sequencing. It can be identified to the sea lion swimming style. It's very effective to swim through narrow underwater places.

Undulatory Swimming

Swimming hydrodynamics have significantly applied BCF (body-caudal fin swimming) to techniques. In addition research on undulatory motion, undulatory Body-caudal fin anguilliform, and undulatory Median-paired fin give interesting conclusions. These natural modes are seen as an alternative to BCF techniques introducing some missing elements as buoyancy, gliding and floating to complement the scale of man's hydrodynamics.

The study draws a conclusion from hydrodynamic properties of cephalopods as implied to human kinetics, discerning significant patterns, like floating, puddle, undulation or efficiency. In biomechanical aspect medusoid and anguilliform shows positive results: low Reynolds number, low viscous forces, stability, great laminar flow, linear momentum and efficient velocity.

Lifesaving Strokes

- Lifesaving stroke: Similar to the side stroke, but only the bottom arm moves while the top arm tows a swimmer in distress.
- Lifesaving approach stroke (also known as *head-up front crawl* or *Tarzan stroke*): Similar to the front crawl, but with the eyes to the front above the water level, such as to observe the surroundings as for example a swimmer in distress or a ball.
- Pushing rescue stroke: This stroke helps to assist a tired swimmer: The tired swimmer lies on the back and the rescuer swims a breaststroke kick and pushes against the soles of the tired swimmer.

- Pulling rescue stroke: This stroke helps to assist a swimmer in distress. Both swimmers lie on the back, and the rescuer grabs the armpits of the swimmer in distress and performs a breaststroke kick (on the back) for forwarding motion. The kick has to be not too shallow as otherwise the victim will be hit.
- Extended Arm Tow (unconscious victim): swimming sidestroke or breaststroke on their back, the rescuer holds the head with a straight arm, the hand cupping underneath the chin, and ensures that the mouth and nose are out of the water.
- Arm Tow: the rescuer swims sidestroke, behind the casualty holds the upper right arm of a casualty with their left hand or vice versa, lifting the casualty out of the water.
- Vice Grip Turn and Trawl: used on a victim with a suspected spinal injury. The lifeguard approaches slowly to the victim (who is usually face down in water), places one hand on the victim's chin, with arm pressed firmly against the victim's chest. The other hand is placed on the back of the victim's head with the arm down the victim's back. Both arms press together (like a vice), and the lifeguard uses his feet to begin moving forward and then rolls under the victim to come up alongside her or him, but with the victim now on his or her back. (This is one of the hardest lifesaving maneuvers, as the grip must be perfect on the first attempt; otherwise, the victim may be given further spinal damage, such as paralysis.)
- Clothes swimming: The swimmer is wearing clothes that restrict movement when wet, i.e. almost all clothes. This is done to practice situations where the swimmer fell in the water dressed or the rescuer did not have time to undress. Due to the restricted movement and the weight of wet clothes out of the water, an overarm recovery is not possible. Most swimmers swim breaststroke, but any stroke with underwater recovery is feasible.
- Rescue tube swimming: The lifeguard pulls a flotation device, which is pushed forward when approaching the victim.

Composite Stroke

The most famous and transient variant of the composite stroke, a stroke composed of two or more basic strokes, is the US combat sidestroke, developed by United States Navy Seal's. Further variants are the elaboration of this basic composite method.

- Basic composite is change or switch between two basic strokes, composite is just switch-between, for instance Side to Breast Composite, Over arm 1 Arm Lead Flutter kick to Front crawl flutter/scissor is switch-between with one switch-in, change between sidestroke and switch-in breaststroke as to change between two basic strokes.
- Composite I is switch-between one switch-in, Composite II, is switch-between two switch-ins, switch between two different basic switch-in strokes, Over arm 1 Arm Lead Flutter kick to 2 Arms Lead Dolphin, switch-between implies switch with flip drill, 1 arm to 2 arms lead, so it is composite spin, or switch-between flip, Over arm 1 Arm Lead Scissor kick to Front crawl flutter/scissor, is change with spin advanced or composite as switch-between where we have spin advancing from scissor to flutter/scissor kick, which is legs flip from

basic to switch-between kick, or improved flip kick, In-II, Front crawl flutter/scissor Dolphin/Dolphin flutter, switch-in between two switch-ins, change of two switch-ins within one basic stroke, In-I switch of non-switch-in and switch-in within one basic stroke, switch-between 2 switch-ins, switch-in 2 switch-ins, Floating Flutter/Scissor to 2 Arm Lead Frog/Scissor 2 Arms Lead Dolphin/Flutter, two switch-in, Comp II switch-between 2 switch-between,

- Composite III, switch-between 3 switch-ins, and In could be flip (spin), advanced flip (spin), ½ stroke is float stroke in combination with different legs drill, Composite IV, switch-between 4 switch-ins, change of 2 switch-ins within two basic strokes, In-IV, switch-in between 4 switch-in, change between 4 switch-ins within one basic stroke,
- Half Composite, switch-between two half strokes, ½ Composite V, Easy ½ stroke, switch-in between colchian element and float, easy switch-in drill is combination of ½ stroke and float, switch-in of ½ stroke come as spin, if switch between non-switch-in and switch-ins (or switch-in and switch-ins) then as advanced flip, 2 Arms Lead Flutter to 2 Arms Lead Flutter/Frog is advanced spin, or 2 Arms Lead Flutter to 2 Arms Lead Flutter/Frog/Dolphin, 0-2 advanced flip, 2 Arms Lead Flutter/Frog to 2 Arms Lead Flutter/Frog/Dolphin, 1-2 advanced flip, 2 Composite, switch-between switch-betweens, implying switch of four basic strokes,
- 1½ Composite, switch of three basic strokes, switch-in of drill, and switch-in of element, switch of drill is switch-in, whereas switch of an element is ½ switch-in, spin, switch of arm or leg work out.

Where as switch-in is composite of drills withing one basic stroke, and switch-between is composite of drills withing two or more basic strokes.

Without Forward Motion

- Survival floating (also known as *dead man float* and drownproofing): Lying on the prone (face down in water) with minimal leg movement, and staying afloat with the natural buoyancy. Lift the head to breathe only then back to floating. This style is only to stay afloat and to rest.
- Back floating: Similar to the survival floating, except on the back.
- Treading water: The swimmer is in the water head up and feet down. Different kicks, such as the eggbeater kick, and hand movements are used to stay afloat. This is useful to keep the head out of the water for a better view or to catch an object as for example in water polo.
- Sculling: This is a figure 8 movement of the hands for forward motion or upward lift. Used in surf lifesaving, water polo, synchronized swimming and treading water.
- Turtle float: The knees are raised to the chest and encircled by the arms.
- Jellyfish float: Holding the ankles with the hands.
- Head first surface dive

Front Crawl

The front crawl is a classic swimming stroke and is usually one of the first learned when you take swimming lessons. The front crawl is also known as freestyle swimming, and is the fastest of all the swimming strokes, The front crawl is a basic swimming stroke, but it still requires a good deal of timing, coordination and technique for it to be effective.

Front Crawl Swimming Technique

Have a Neutral Head Position

In the past, it was often advised to lift the head up and to look forward while swimming front crawl. The idea is that by lifting the head higher up in the water, less drag is created resulting in faster swimming times. However, there are two problems with that approach:

1. Your hips and legs often have the tendency to drop when you lift your head up. As a consequence, you create more drag instead of less. Furthermore you need to kick harder to keep your hips and legs up.

2. If you look forward at all times while swimming front crawl, you put your neck in an awkward position which can lead to neck injuries over the course of several years.

It is best to keep your head in line with your trunk in a neutral position and look straight down. This helps you to keep your body horizontal in the water, creates the least amount of drag and also prevents neck injuries.

It may still be necessary to look forward from time to time to avoid obstacles or to orient yourself. As long as you keep this to a minimum this shouldn't be a problem. An alternative is to look slightly forward but *with your eyes only*.

Be Balanced and Roll your Body

While you swim freestyle, you should aim to keep your body as horizontal as possible in the water. This is called being balanced. When you are balanced you will create the least amount of drag. And as explained above, a correct head position has a big influence on your balance.

When you swim front crawl, you should let your body roll freely from side to side, following the movements of your arms. Swimmers often have the tendency to roll too little rather than too much. Rolling from side to side allows you to engage large muscle groups (chest, back, abs in addition to shoulders and legs) and consequently improves your propulsion.

While your body rolls from side to side, your head should remain static, looking straight down, except when breathing, as described next.

Roll to Breathe

To breathe in, you roll farther on your side than during the non-breathing arm strokes. Your head simply follows along your body then rolls a little bit farther until your mouth clears the water so you can inhale. You should roll your head as little as is needed because rolling too much can also disrupt balance and strain your neck.

In fact, if you watch the pros swim, you will see that they inhale with their mouth slightly to the side and in the trough of the bow wave created by their head, so that they need to rotate their head as little as possible. While they do this, typically one lens of their swimming goggles is underwater and one lens above water. However, being able to do this takes a lot of practice.

A common error less experienced swimmers do is that they lift their head first before they roll on their side to breathe. As explained above, this disrupts balance and causes their hips and legs to drop, increasing drag.

The Muscles used in a Front Crawl

Upper Body

Freestyle is performed by using an alternating arm motion to move a swimmer through the water. As one arm moves from the hips to the head out of the water, the other arm does an S-curve pull under the water. This S-curve pull uses most of the muscles in the upper body. The first part of the S-curve – where the hand catches the water and begins the pull by executing a sculling motion – uses the forearm muscles and your latissimus dorsi. The middle portion of the S-curve pull works the biceps and deltoids, while the completion of the curve – the portion where the arm leaves the water – works the triceps. Throughout the pull, the pectoral muscles are engaged, as are the hand muscles, which must remain tight to keep the fingers together to increase the force of the pull.

Lower Body

Freestyle swimmers use a flutter kick to propel themselves through the water. The flutter kick uses alternating movements of the feet, pressing one foot down slightly into the water while the other foot returns to the surface. This movement keeps all the major muscle groups in the lower body engaged – including the feet muscles, calf muscles, hamstrings and quads – although the bulk of the movement is generated by the hips. The movement begins with the glutes – the muscles in the buttocks – which power the motion all the way down the legs to the feet.

Torso

The torso plays a key role in generating the power necessary to drive the front crawl. Although the midsection remains straight, it rotates from side to side. As it does, it generates torque, which increases the swimmer's speed. This rotating motion forces the core – specifically the abdominal and oblique muscles – to be engaged and stabilize the swimmer's body in the water. The back muscles, including the spinus erectors, are also engaged during this rotation.

Muscle Injuries

Improper alignment, or putting too much stress on a muscle, leads to most of the injuries related to the front crawl. Failure to keep the body straight – from the tip of the head to the tailbone – leads to injuries of the neck and lower back muscles. Keeping the toes unnaturally pointed during the flutter kick causes a condition called plantar flexion, which leads to cramps in the calves. Putting too much stress on the deltoids – the shoulder muscles – by using pull buoys or arm paddles causes swimmer's shoulder, an injury characterized by fatigued muscles and overstretched or inflamed tendons.

Trudgen

Trudgen, swimming style that is performed with alternate armor over the water as in the crawl and scissors park with the legs. The style is named after the British swimmer John Trudgen (1852-1903) who had learned it in South America and introduced it to European competition refuge in the 1870s. Around 1900 replaced by crawl.

To master the trudgen stroke, combine the arm action of the crawl or freestyle stroke with the leg action of side stroke (scissor kick).

Start in a Face-down Glide Position

Begin the crawl stroke with just your arms: Swing your arms from your shoulders, first one, then the other, with one arm recovering while the other strokes. Each hand knifes through the water, then sweeps down and back to your side, pushing water toward your feet.

Straighten your arm to push water back, then bend your elbow to lift and swing your arm back to the forward position.

Roll your lower body slightly, letting one hip drop below the other (whichever side feels more comfortable to you). If your left hip drops, breathe on the right side, and vice versa.

As your right arm leaves the water, take a breath.

Snap your legs together, like scissors closing, as your right arm re-enters the water.

Keep legs together and motionless as you sweep your left arm through the water. When your right arm enters the water for a new cycle, repeat the scissor kick.

Butterfly Stroke

The butterfly stroke is one of the fastest competitive swimming strokes. And though it is difficult to master, it is fun. After all, who doesn't want to swim like a dolphin – intermittently flying above the water and plunging right back into the blue! Doing it regularly will make you fit, toned, increase your strength, improve heart health, and decrease cholesterol.

The butterfly stroke is also called "the fly" by swimmers. It is swum on the chest, with both the arms moving simultaneously to displace the water and the legs kicking to propel the body forward. This coordinated whole body movement will help you move faster than the freestyle stroke.

Elements of a Fast Butterfly

Quick, early catch.

Just like in freestyle where you want to have an early vertical forearm, so it is with the butterfly. Beginner butterfliers will be tempted to pull straight down towards the bottom of the pool in order to bring their head above the water.

Focus point:Finger tips down, palms backwards.

Relaxed recovery.

This requires flexibility in the shoulders, chest and back. What happens when you start to fatigue? Your arms and shoulders seize, and you begin to experience what swimmers know as "T-rex'ing"–where your arms lose it's relaxed, Gumby-like posture and they bend and harden, shortening your stroke.

Charge forwards; not up and down.

When learning butterfly most swimmers tend to swim in an exaggerated wave pattern. They pull their heads straight-up in order to breathe, and then dive straight back down. This leads to a lot of wasted effort. When breathing and pulling through the water your focus should always be on swimming forwards.

Skim your chin across the surface of the water.

When you watch Michael Phelps breathe you notice how low of a profile he keeps when breathing–this isn't an accident. He picks up his head as much as he needs to in order to take a breath, in no higher. This results in less wasted energy, increased efficiency, and less of the up-and-down bobbing that is so common with an inefficient fly stroke.

Two kicks per pull.

The butterfly kick has a few different functions within the overall stroke–it helps to create a little bit of propulsion, assists in creating lift to allow the swimmer to pick their head up out of the water (first kick of the stroke cycle), while the second kick drives the arms and hands forward into the catch phase of the pull.

Speed and Ergonomics

The peak speed of the butterfly is faster than that of the front crawl, or freestyle due to the synchronous pull/push with both arms and legs, which is done quite fast. Yet since speed drops significantly during the recovery phase, it is overall slightly slower than front crawl, especially over longer distances. Another reason it is slower is because of the extremely different physical exertion it puts on the swimmer compared to the freestyle. Its name was taken from the butterfly.

The breaststroke, backstroke, and front crawl can all be swum easily even if the swimmer's technique is flawed. The butterfly, however, is unforgiving of mistakes in style; it is very difficult to overcome a poor butterfly technique with brute strength. Many swimmers and coaches consider it the most difficult swimming style. The main difficulty for beginners is the synchronous over-water recovery, especially when combined with breathing, since both arms, the head, shoulders and part of the chest have to be lifted out of the water for these tasks. Once efficient technique has been developed, it becomes a smooth, fast stroke.

Technique

The butterfly technique with the dolphin kick consists of synchronous arm movement with a synchronous leg kick. Good technique is crucial to swim this style effectively. The wave-like body movement is also very significant in creating propulsion, as this is the key to easy synchronous over-water recovery and breathing.

In the initial position, the swimmer lies on the breast, the arms are stretched to the front, and the legs are extended to the back.

Arm Movement

The butterfly stroke has three major parts, the pull, the push, and the recovery. These can also be further subdivided. From the initial position, the arm movement starts very similarly to the breast stroke. At the beginning the hands sink a little bit down with the palms facing outwards and slightly down at shoulder width, then the hands move out to create a Y. This is called catching the water. The pull movement follows a semicircle with the elbow higher than the hand and the hand pointing towards the center of the body and downward to form the traditionally taught "keyhole".

The push pushes the palm backward through the water underneath the body at the beginning and at the side of the body at the end of the push. The swimmer only pushes the arms 1/3 of the way to the hips, making it easier to enter into the recovery and making the recovery shorter and making the breathing window shorter. The movement increases speed throughout the pull-push phase until the hand is the fastest at the end of the push. This step is called the release and is crucial for the recovery. The speed at the end of the push is used to help with the recovery.

The recovery swings the arms sideways across the water surface to the front, with the elbows straight. The arms should be swung forward from the end of the underwater movement, the extension of the triceps in combination with the butterfly kick will allow the arm to be brought forwards relaxed yet quickly. In contrast to the front crawl recovery, this arm recovery is a ballistic shot. The only other way of lifting the arms and the shoulders out of the water is by dropping one's hip. Therefore, the recovery, at least the acceleration of the arms, is in no way relaxed. It is important not to enter the water too early, because this would generate extra resistance as the arms moved forward in the water against the swimming direction, however, during longer distances, this cannot be avoided, and it is more important to avoid dropping one's hips. A high elbow recovery, as in front crawl, would be disadvantageous because of the natural undulations that are partially caused by the recovery and the relaxed movement caused by the momentum of a triceps extension. Limitations of the shoulder movement in the human body make such a motion unlikely. Hands should enter into the water again at 11 and one with thumbs entering first and pinkies last.

The arms enter the water with the thumbs first at shoulder width. A wider entry loses movement in the next pull phase, and a smaller entry, where the hands touch, wastes energy. The cycle repeats with the pull phase. However, some people prefer to touch in front, because it helps them catch water, as long as they can do this efficiently, they are not losing anything.

Leg Movement

The legs are synchronized with each other which uses a whole different set of muscles. The shoulders are brought above the surface by a strong up and medium down kick, and back below the surface by a strong down and up kick. A smooth undulation fuses the motion together.

The feet are pressed together to avoid loss of water pressure. The feet are naturally pointing downwards, giving downwards thrust, moving up the feet and pressing down the head.

There is no actual stipulation in competitive butterfly rules that a swimmer make a fixed number of pulses in butterfly–the swimmer may kick as little or as much as he or she may wish. While competitive rules allow such a choice, the typical method of swimming butterfly is with two kicks.

As butterfly originated as a variant on breaststroke, it would be performed with a breaststroke or whip kick by some swimmers. While breaststroke was separated from butterfly in 1953, the breaststroke kick in butterfly was not officially outlawed until 2001. However a number of Masters swimmers were upset with the change since they came from a time when butterfly was usually swum with a breaststroke kick. FINA was then convinced to allow a breaststroke kick in Masters swimming. Given the option, most swimmers choose to use a dolphin kicking action, but there still is a small minority of swimmers who prefer the breaststroke kick, for recreational swimming and even for competition.

Breathing

There is only a short window for breathing in the butterfly. If this window is missed, swimming becomes very difficult. Optimally, a butterfly swimmer synchronizes the taking of breaths with the undulation of the body to simplify the breathing process; doing this well requires some attention to butterfly stroke technique. The breathing process begins during the underwater "press" portion of the stroke. As the hands and forearms move underneath the chest, the body will naturally rise toward the surface of the water. With minimum effort, the swimmer can lift the head to fully break the surface. The swimmer breathes in through the mouth. The head goes back in the water after the arms come out of the water as they are swinging forward over the surface of the water. If the head stays out too long, the recovery is hindered. The swimmer breathes out through mouth and nose till the next breath.

Normally, a breath is taken every other stroke. This can be sustained over long distances. Often, breathing every stroke slows the swimmer down. (At a certain level, a breathing stroke becomes just as fast as a nonbreathing stroke; therefore, very experienced competitors, such as Michael Phelps, may breathe every stroke.) Other intervals of breathing practised by elite swimmers include the "two up, one down" approach in which the swimmer breathes for two successive strokes and then keeps their head in the water on the next stroke, which is easier on the lungs. Swimmers with good lung capacity might also breathe every 3rd stroke during sprints for the finish. Some swimmers can even hold their breaths for an entire race (assuming that it is a short one). To be able to swim with best results it is important to keep one's head down when taking a breath. If the swimmer lifts his or her head too high the swimmer's hips often drop, creating drag, thus slowing the swimmer down. The closer one's head is to the water the better one swim is the general technique used by swimmers.

Body Movement

Swimming butterfly is difficult if the core is not utilized, and correct timing and body movement makes swimming butterfly much easier. The body moves in a wave-like fashion, controlled by the core, and as the chest is pressed down, the hips go up, and the posterior breaks the water surface and transfers into a fluid kick. During the push phase, the chest goes up and the hips are at their lowest position. In this style, the second pulse in the cycle is stronger than the first pulse, as the second pulse is more in flow with the body movement.

Although butterfly is very compatible with diving, the resulting reduction in wave drag does not lead to an overall reduction of drag. In the modern style of the butterfly stroke one does only little vertical movement of the body.

Start

Butterfly uses the regular start for swimming. After the start a gliding phase follows under water, followed by dolphin kicks swim under water. Swimming under water reduces the drag from breaking the surface and is very economical. Rules allow for 15 m of underwater swimming before the head must break the surface, and regular swimming begins.

Turn and Finish

During turns and during the finish, both hands must simultaneously touch the wall while the swimmer remains swimming face down. The swimmer touches the wall with both hands while bending the elbows slightly. The bent elbows allow the swimmer to push himself or herself away from the wall and turn sideways. One hand leaves the wall to be moved to the front underwater. At the same time the legs are pulled closer and moved underneath of the body towards the wall. The second hand leaves the wall to be moved to the front over water. It is commonly referred to as an "over/under turn" or an "open turn". The legs touch the wall and the hands are at the front. The swimmer sinks under water and lies on the breast, or nearly so. Then the swimmer pushes off the wall, keeping a streamline position with the hands to the front. Similar to the start, the swimmer is allowed to swim 15 m underwater before the head must break the surface. Most swimmers dolphin kick after an initial gliding phase.

The finish requires the swimmer to touch the wall with both hands at the same time, in the same horizontal plane.

Styles

There are four styles of butterfly stroke.

Two main styles of butterfly stroke seen today are: "arm pull up simultaneous with dolphin kick" and "arm pull down simultaneous with dolphin kick".

"Arm pull up simultaneous with dolphin kick": After head goes underwater, both arms go underwater but still higher than head. After first dolphin kick, *pull both arms immediately with downward motion*. While pulling arms, legs are relaxed, both knees and waist are slightly bent to prepare dolphin kick. After arms push water backward, pull arms up simultaneous with dolphin kick. In this style, turning point from drowning to floating is at the time of downward arm motion.

"Arm pull down simultaneous with dolphin kick": After head goes underwater, both arms go underwater until lower than head. After first dolphin kick, *raise both arms with relax*. While rising arms, bend both knees and waist to send body back to the surface and prepare dolphin kick. Pull both arms downward while executing dolphin kick. After this sequence, immediately push the water backward. In this style, turning point from drowning to floating is at the time of waist bend.

Two additional styles of butterfly stroke are similar to the two styles above, but without a "second" dolphin kick. This allows the swimmer to conserve energy and be more relaxed.

Breaststroke

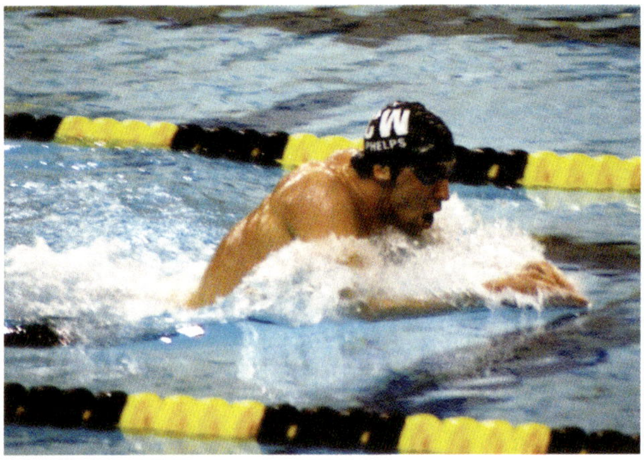

A breaststroke at the Missouri Grand Prix.

Breaststroke is a swimming style in which the swimmer is on their chest and the torso does not rotate. It is the most popular recreational style due to the swimmer's head being out of the water a large portion of the time, and that it can be swum comfortably at slow speeds. In most swimming classes, beginners learn either the breaststroke or the front crawl first. However, at the competitive level, swimming breaststroke at speed requires comparable endurance and strength to other strokes. Some people refer to breaststroke as the "frog" stroke, as the arms and legs move somewhat like a frog swimming in the water. The stroke itself is the slowest of any competitive strokes and is thought to be the oldest of all swimming strokes.

Speed and Ergonomics

Breaststroke is the slowest of the four official styles in competitive swimming. The fastest breaststrokers can swim about 1.70 metres per second. It is sometimes the hardest to teach to rising swimmers after butterfly due to the importance of timing and the coordination required to move the legs properly.

In the breaststroke, the swimmer leans on the chest, arms breaking the surface of the water slightly, legs always underwater and the head underwater for the second half of the stroke. The kick is sometimes referred to as a "frog kick" because of the resemblance to the movement of a frog's hind legs; however, when done correctly it is more of a "whip kick" due to the whip-like motion that moves starting at the core down through the legs.

The body is often at a steep angle to the forward movement, which slows down the swimmer more than any other style. Professional breaststrokers use abdominal muscles and hips to add extra power to the kick, although most do not perfect this technique until the collegiate level. This much faster form of breaststroke is referred to as "wave-action" breaststroke and fully incorporates the whip-kick.

A special feature of competitive breaststroke is the underwater pullout. From the streamline position, one uses the arms to pull all the way down past the hips. As the arms are pulling down, one downward dolphin kick is allowed (as of the 2005 season), though still optional; more than one dolphin kick will result in disqualification. This is followed by the recovery of the arms to the streamline position once more with a breaststroke kick. The pullout is also called the "pull down". The pullout at the start and after the turns contributes significantly to the swimming times. Open turns can be easily performed at the walls, but both hands must make contact with the wall. Therefore, one way to improve swimming times is to focus on the start and the turns.

Technique

The breaststroke starts with the swimmer lying in the water face down, arms extended straight forward and legs extended straight to the back.

Arm Movement

There are three steps to the arm movement: outsweep, insweep, and recovery. The movement starts with the outsweep. From the streamline position, the palms turn out and the hands separate to slightly past shoulder width. The outsweep is followed by the insweep, where the hands point down and push the water backwards. The elbows stay in the horizontal plane through the shoulders. The hands push back until approximately the vertical plane through the shoulders. At the end of the insweep the hands come together with facing palms in front of the chest and the elbows are at the side at the body. In the recovery phase, the hands are moved forward again into the initial position under water. The entire arm stroke starts slowly, increases speed to the peak arm movement speed in the insweep phase, and slows down again during recovery. The goal is to produce maximum thrust during the insweep phase, and minimum drag during the recovery phase. Another variant is the underwater pull-down, similar to the push phase of a butterfly stroke. This stroke continues the insweep phase and pushes the hands all the way to the back to the sides of the hip. This greatly increases the push froAs a variant, it is possible to recover the arms over water. This reduces drag, but requires more power. Some competitive swimmers use this variant in competition.≤ m one stroke, but also makes recovery more difficult. This style is well suited for underwater swimming. However, FINA allows this stroke only for the first stroke after the start and each turn. In late 2005, FINA has also introduced a new rule which allows you to perform a single downward kick after the push off the wall.

Leg Movement

The leg movement, colloquially known as the "frog kick" or "whip kick", consists of two phases: bringing the feet into position for the thrust phase and the insweep phase. From the initial position with the legs stretched out backward, the feet are moved together towards the posterior, while the knees stay together. The knees should not sink too low, as this increases the drag. Then the feet point outward in preparation for the thrust phase. In the thrust phase, the legs are moved elliptically back to the initial position. During this movement, the knees are kept together. The legs move slower while bringing the legs into position for the thrust phase, and move very fast during the thrust phase. Again, the goal is to produce maximum thrust during the insweep phase, and minimise drag during the recovery phase. In the recovery phase the lower leg and the feet are in the wake of the upper leg, and the feet are pointed to the rear. In the thrust phase all three parts create their own wake, and the flat end of the feet acts like a hydrofoil aligned to give maximum forward thrust. The resulting drag coefficient (or more precisely the frontal area) is thus doubled in the thrust phase.

A fit adult creates a wake. Drag due to a wake is Newtonian drag, increasing with the square of the velocity. For example, if the relative speed between the water and the leg is twice as high on the thrust phase than on the recovery phase, the thrust is four times as high as the drag. Assuming the legs are recovered with a relative speed between leg and body which amounts to the same as the relative speed between water and body, the legs must be kicked back with five times the mean velocity of the swimmer. This limits the top speed. Both effects together, velocity and frontal area, yield a thrust-to-drag ratio of 8 for the legs.

As a variant, some swimmers move the knees apart during the preparation phase and keep them apart until almost the end of the thrust phase. Moving both knee and foot outwards like a real frog avoids the extreme rotation in the lower leg.

All other variants fail to increase the frontal area, yet swimmers using them still generate some thrust by the velocity variation and do not drown. Another variant of the breaststroke kick is the scissor kick, however, this kick violates the rules of the FINA as it is no longer symmetrical. Swimming teachers put a great effort into steering the students away from the scissor kick. In the scissor kick, one leg moves as described above, but the other leg does not form an elliptical movement but merely an up-down movement similar to the flutter kick of front crawl. Some swimming teachers believe that learning the front crawl first gives a higher risk of an incorrect scissor kick when learning breaststroke afterwards.

Breaststroke can also be swum with the dolphin kick in butterfly, but this also violates the FINA rules. One kick is allowed, however, at the start and at the turn, providing that it is part of the body's natural movement.

The harmonic movements of the dolphin kick and flutter kick are in contrast to the breaststroke whip kick, which really deserves the name kick. Scissor kick and frog kick are intermediate. Humans have strong muscles in the legs and would need swim fins (like a frog) to bring all their power into the water and stand with the sole of the feet on the water. Rather the leg grabs almost as much water as the foot and a small amount of water is accelerated to high kinetic energy, but not much impulse is transferred. The toes are bent, the feet point 45° outwards, the sole points backwards, to mimic a hydrofoil. While closing in a V shape to the rear a small "lifting" force can be felt. Unlike in the other kicks, the joints are moved into extrema. Before the kick the knee is maximally bent and the upper leg is rotating along its axis to its extreme outer position and the lower leg is twisted to extreme, at the end of the kick the ankles are maximally turned to the inside so that the soles clap together to achieve a nozzle effect like in a jelly fish. Therefore, training involves getting flexible in addition to fitness and precision. The sudden sideways stress on knee at the kick can lead to uncomfortable noise and feeling for the beginner and to wear for the senior.

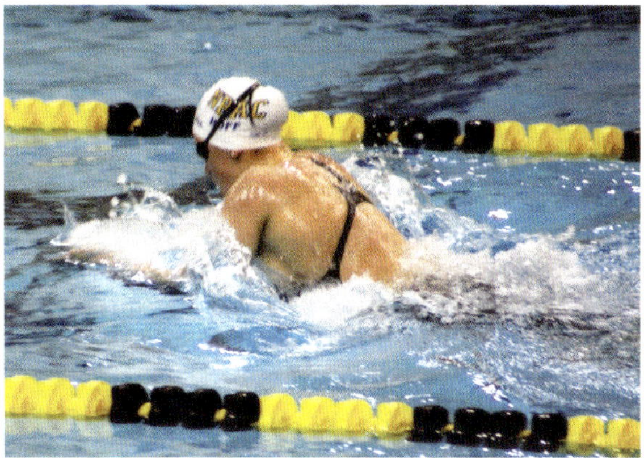

Breaststroke at Missouri Grand Prix.

Breathing

The easiest way to breathe during breaststroke is to let the head follow the spine. When the swimmer's elbows have reached the line of his eye and have begun to rise, his head starts to lift. If he uses his high elbows as a hinge for the inward sweep of his hands and forearms, he will create the leverage he needs to use his abdominal muscles to bring his hips forward. When his hips move forward, his chest, shoulders and upper back will automatically lift up. Breathing is usually done during the beginning of the insweep phase of the arms, and the swimmer breathes in ideally through the mouth. The swimmer breathes out through mouth and nose during the recovery and gliding phase. Breaststroke can be swum faster if submerged completely, but FINA requires the head to break the surface once per cycle except for the first cycle after the start and each turn. Thus, competitive swimmers usually make one underwater pull-out, pushing the hands all the way to the back after the start and each turn.

Recreational swimmers often keep their head above water at all times when they swim breaststroke.

Body Movement

The movement starts in the initial position with the body completely straight, body movement is coordinated such that the legs are ready for the thrust phase while the arms are halfway through the insweep, and the head is out of the water for breathing. In this position the body has also the largest angle to the horizontal. The arms are recovered during the thrust phase of the legs. After the stroke the body is kept in the initial position for some time to utilize the gliding phase. Depending on the distance and fitness the duration of this gliding phase varies. Usually the gliding phase is shorter during sprints than during long distance swimming. The gliding phase is also longer during the underwater stroke after the start and each turn. However, the gliding phase is usually the longest phase in one entire cycle of breaststroke.

Start

Breaststroke uses the regular start for swimming. Some swimmers use a variant called the frog start, where the legs are pulled forward sharply before being extended again quickly during the airborne phase of the start. After the start a gliding phase follows under water, followed by one underwater pulldown and dolphin kick, then one whip kick as the hands are recovered back to a streamline. This is known as the pull-out. The head must break the surface before the arms reach their widest point on the first stroke after the pull-out. The downward butterfly kick was legalized by FINA, WWF and the NCAA in 2005, and remains optional. The downward fly kick is now allowed in MCSL.

Turn and Finish

For competitive swimming it is important that the wall at the end of the lane is always touched by both hands (known as a "Two-Hand Touch") at the same time due to FINA regulations.

The turn is initiated by touching the wall during the gliding or during the recovery phase of the arms, depending on how the wall can be touched faster. After touching the wall, the legs are pulled underneath of the body. The body turns sideways while one hand is moved forward (i.e. towards the head) along the side of the body. When the body is almost completely turned, the other hand will be swung straight up through the air such that both hands meet at the front at the same time. At that time the body should also be almost in the horizontal and partially or totally submerged. After the body is completely submerged, the body is pushed off the wall with both legs. Doing this under water will reduce the drag. After a gliding phase, an underwater pull-out is done, followed by another gliding phase and then regular swimming. The head must break the surface during the second stroke.

As a variant, some swimmers experiment with a flip over turn similar to front crawl. The finish is similar to the touching of the wall during a turn.

Styles

The three main styles of breaststroke seen today are the conventional (flat), undulating, and wave-style. The undulating style is usually swum by extremely flexible swimmers, (e.g. Amanda Beard), and few people have the flexibility to accomplish it. The wave-style breaststroke was pioneered by Hungarian Swimming Coach Joseph Nagy. The breaststroke style was swum and made famous by Mike Barrowman when he set a world record using it, is now commonly swum by Olympians, though Australian swimmers, most prominently Leisel Jones, generally seem to shun it. Olympian Ed Moses still swims a more flat- style, despite the rapidly increasing popularity of the wave-style.

The wave-style breaststroke starts in a streamlined position, with shoulders shrugged to decrease drag in the water. While the conventional style is strongest at the outsweep, the wave-style puts much emphasis on the insweep, thus making the head rise later than in the conventional style. The wave-style pull is a circular motion with the hands accelerating to maximum speed and recovering in front of the chin, elbows staying at the surface and in front of the shoulders at all times. The high elbows creates the leverage for the powerful torso and abdominal muscles to assist in the stroke. During the insweep, the swimmer accelerates their hands and hollows their back and lifts themself out of the water to breathe. To visualize, some say that the hands anchor themselves in the water while the hips thrust forward.

The hollowed back and accelerating hands would lift the head out of the water. The head stays in a natural position, looking down and forward, and the swimmer inhales at this point. The feet retract to the bottom without moving the thigh, thus reducing resistance. The swimmer is at their highest point at this point.

Then the swimmer shrugs their shoulders and throws their arms and shoulders forward, lunging cat-like back into the water (though the emphasis is to go *forward*, not down). As the swimmer sinks, they arch their back, and kicks. Timing is very important in order for the kick to transfer all of its force via the arched back, but the optimum time is when the arms are 3/4 extended. Then the swimmer kicks and presses on their chest, undulating a little underwater, and squeezing the gluteus maximus to prevent the legs and feet from rising out of the water. The swimmer has now returned to the streamlined position, and the cycle starts again.

Incidentally, the wave motion should not be overly emphasized and the swimmer should only rise until the water reaches his biceps, instead of pushing his entire torso out of the water, wasting a great deal of energy.

Benefits of Breast Stroke

Swimming Breaststroke

Breaststroke will take time to perfect, but the basics are easy to grasp. During the pull, the hands and arms should press out in front of the chest in a heart-shaped pattern and recover under the surface of the water. The kick, often referred to as the frog or whip kick, is a simultaneous circular motion under the water, similar to the action of a frog. During the stroke, for every one kick, one pull should also be executed, and it should done in the following pattern: pull, breath, kick, glide.

Lower Body Benefits

Breaststroke is a stroke that requires a strong kick to propel the body through the water. As the feet move out and away from the body, it promotes hip, knee, and foot flexibility as your feet are flexed and pointed out. The feet should stay wider than the knees throughout the kick. The muscles used throughout the kick are similar to other kicks. The breaststroke kick also engages the inner and outer thigh muscles that are not used as often in other strokes.

Upper Body Benefits

Breaststroke is an overall upper body workout. This stroke will strengthen the muscles your upper body but will engage the forearm, chest and upper back muscles more than any other stroke. The outward sweeping motion of the hands and inward pull of the water toward the breast requires use of the deltoids, biceps, triceps, pectorals and trapezius muscles. The faster you swim breaststroke and the more challenging your swim, the stronger these muscles will become.

Core Body Benefits

Freestyle and backstroke are long axis strokes, while breaststroke and butterfly are considered short axis strokes. Breaststroke requires the body to move or bend along the short axis of the body at the hips. During breaststroke, your body should make a wavelike motion, which is the result of the constant upward and downward movement of the chest. Because of this bending wavelike movement, your core body muscles are engaged. Your hips will assist your breathing and momentum by driving downward and forward. The more breaststroke you swim, the more you engage your core body, and thus the stronger it will become.

Fitness Benefits

Of the four competitive strokes, breaststroke is generally the slowest of the four, but it can be swum at any effort. You can use breaststroke to swim long, easy workouts, or you can challenge yourself with a hard breaststroke swim. Swimming will increase your overall fitness level, and breaststroke can be your primary means of swimming or an alternate stroke to use when you need a change.

Backstroke

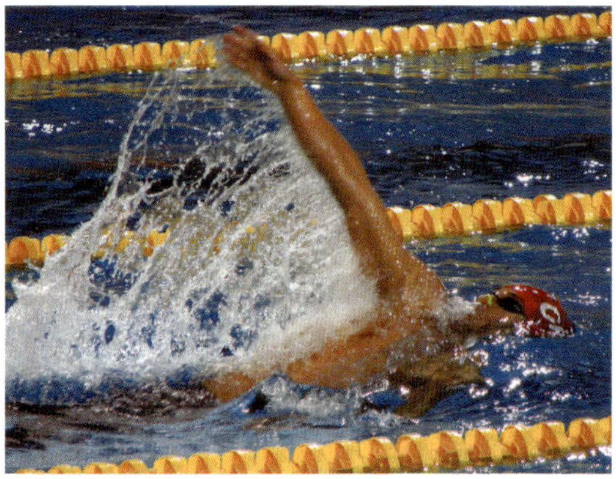

Swimmer doing backstroke at Euros.

Backstroke is one of the four swimming styles used in competitive events regulated by FINA, and the only one of these styles swum on the back. This swimming style has the advantage of easy breathing, but the disadvantage of swimmers not being able to see where they are going. It is also the only competition swimming style that has a different start. The swimming style is similar to an *upside down* front crawl or freestyle. Both backstroke and front crawl are long-axis strokes. In individual medley backstroke is the second style swum; in the medley relay it is the first style swum.

Technique

In the initial position, the swimmer performing backstroke lies flat on the back; arms stretched with extended fingertips, and legs extended backwards.

Arm Movement

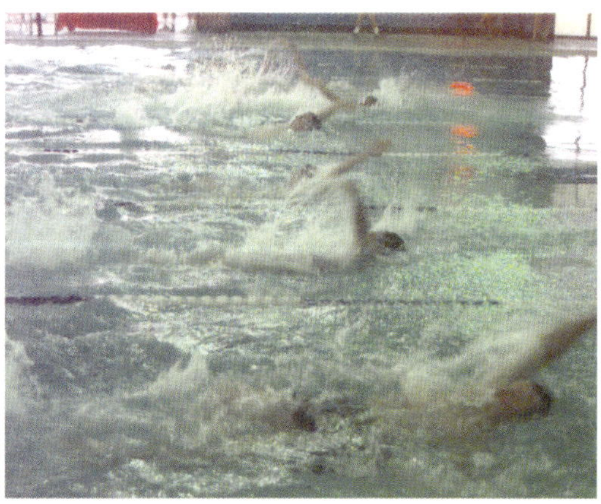

Backstroke swimming (amateur competition, non-optimal style).

In backstroke, the arms contribute most of the forward movement. The arm stroke consists of two main parts: the power phase (consisting of three separate parts) and the recovery. The arms alternate so that always one arm is underwater while the other arm is recovering. One complete arm turn is considered one cycle. From the initial position, one arm sinks slightly under water and turns the palm outward to start the catch phase (first part of the power phase). The hand enters downward (pinkie finger first) then pulling out at a 45 degree angle, catching the water.

During the power phase the hand follows a semi-circular path from the catch to the side of the hip. The palm is always facing away from the swimming direction, while remaining straight as an extension of the arm, and the elbow always points downward towards the bottom of the pool. This is done so that both the arms and the elbow can push the maximum amount of water back in order to push the body forward. At the height of the shoulders, the upper and lower arms should have their maximum angle of about 90 degrees. This is called the Mid-Pull of the power phase.

The Mid-Pull phase consists of pushing the palm of the hand as far down as possible with the fingers pointing upward. Again, the goal is to push the body forward against the water. At the very end of the Mid-Pull, the palm flaps down for a last push forward down to a depth of 45 cm, creating the finish of the power phase. Besides pushing the body forward, this also helps with the rolling back to the other side as part of the body movement. During the power phase, the fingers of the hand can be slightly apart, as this will increase the resistance of the hand in the water due to turbulence.

To prepare for the recovery phase, the hand is rotated so that the palms point towards the legs and the thumb side points upwards. At the beginning of the recovery phase of the one arm, the other arm begins its power phase. The recovering arm is moved in a semicircle straight over the shoulders to the front. During this recovery, the palm rotates so that the small finger enters the water first, allowing for the least amount of resistance, and the palms point outward. After a short gliding phase, the cycle repeats with the preparation for the next power phase.

Variants

A variant is to move both arms synchronized and not alternating, similar to an upside down breast stroke. This is easier to coordinate, and the peak speed during the combined power phase is faster, yet the speed is much slower during the combined recovery. The average speed will usually be less than the average speed of the alternating stroke. This stroke is commonly called the elementary backstroke. This elementary backstroke swim was used in the 1900 and 1908 Olympics. The back-crawl swim supplanted the elementary backstroke swim after 1908 as the competitive back swim and it is now the referred to as the backstroke.

Another variant is the old style of swimming backstroke, where the arm movement formed a complete circle in a windmill type pattern. However, this style is not commonly used for competitive swimming, as a lot of energy is spent on pushing the body up and down instead of forward. Furthermore, the added strain on the shoulder is considered less than ideal and can lead to injuries.

It is also possible to move only one arm at a time, where one arm moves through the power and recovery phases while the other arm rests. This is slow, but it is used frequently to teach students the movement, as they have to concentrate on only one arm.

Leg Movement

The leg movement in backstroke is similar to the flutter kick in front crawl. The kick makes a large contribution to the forward speed, while significantly stabilizing the body.

The leg stroke alternates, with one leg sinking down straight to about 30 degrees. From this position, the leg makes a fast kick upward, slightly bending the knee at the beginning and then stretching it again in the horizontal. However, there are also frequent variants with four or only two kicks per cycle. Usually, sprinters tend to use 6 kicks per cycle, whereas long distance swimmer may use fewer.

Variants

It is also possible to use a butterfly kick, although this is rare except after the initial start and after turns. The dolphin kick is essential for many top athletes because it is the fastest part of the race. It may also constitute the majority of the race (i.e., in the 100 yard backstroke the swimmer may kick underwater dolphin for 15 yards per length which equates to as much as 60 yards kicking in a 100 yd race). A great example of this is Olympic gold medallist Natalie Coughlin. Breaststroke kicks are most comfortable if the arms are used synchronized, as the breaststroke kick makes it more difficult to compensate for the rolling movement with alternating arm cycles. The butterfly kick can be done slightly to one side depending on the rolling motion of the body.

Breathing

Breathing in backstroke is easier than in other strokes, as the mouth and nose are usually above water. Competitive swimmers breathe in through the mouth during the recovery of one arm, and breathe out through the mouth and nose during the pull and push phase of the same arm. This is done to clear the nose of water.

Body Movement

Due to the asynchronous movement of the arms, the body tends to roll around its long axis. By taking advantage of this rolling motion, swimmers can increase their effectiveness while swimming backstroke. The overall position of the body is straight in the horizontal to reduce drag. Beginners frequently let their posterior and thighs sink too low, which increases drag. To avoid this, the upper legs have to be moved to the extreme down position at each kick even with a little help by the back and the foot tips have to be fixed in the extreme lower position and the head is held out of the water to act as a counter-weight.

Start

The backstroke start is the only start from the water. The swimmer faces the wall and grabs part of the start block or the wall with their hands. Ideally, there are grips on the block for this purpose. The legs are placed shoulder width apart on the wall with both heels slightly off the wall. Just before the starting signal, the swimmer pulls their head closer to the start block, while keeping the knees bent at a 90-degree angle. Some swimmers prefer to keep one foot slightly lower than the other during the start.

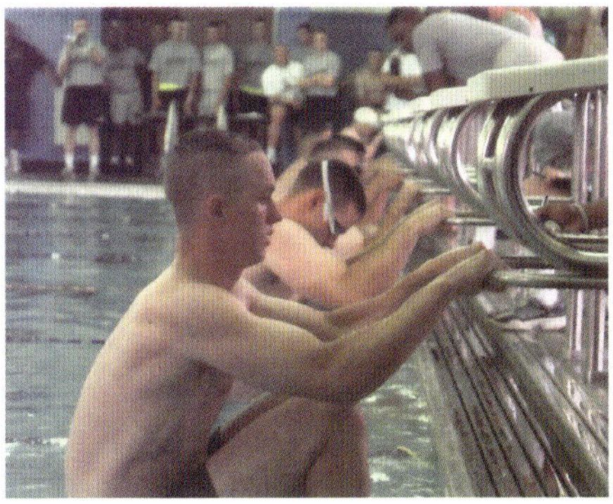

Backstroke start, waiting for the signal.

For the takeoff, the swimmer pushes his or her hands away from the block and swings his or her arms around sideways to the front. At the same time, the swimmer throws his or her head to the back. The swimmer then pushes away from the wall with his feet. Ideally, the swimmer's back is arched during the airborne phase so that only the feet and the hands touch the water while the rest of the body is above the water line. This reduces drag and permits a faster start. On September 21, 2005, FINA modified the backstroke start rule regarding toes below the water line. The feet can now be above the water, but not above or curled over the lip of the pool gutter.

After the start, the swimmer is completely underwater. Due to increased resistance at the surface, experienced swimmers usually swim faster underwater than at the surface. Therefore, most experienced swimmers in backstroke competitions stay under water up to the limit set by FINA (15 meters after the start and after every turn). Most swimmers use a butterfly kick underwater, as this provides more forward movement than the flutter kick. The underwater phase includes the risk of water entering the nose, so most swimmers breathe out through the nose to stop water from entering.

The swimmer's head must break the surface before 15 m under FINA rules. The swimmer starts swimming with one arm, followed by the other arm with half a cycle delay. The swimmer continues in regular swimming style, staying on the back for the entire time except the turns.

Turn and Finish

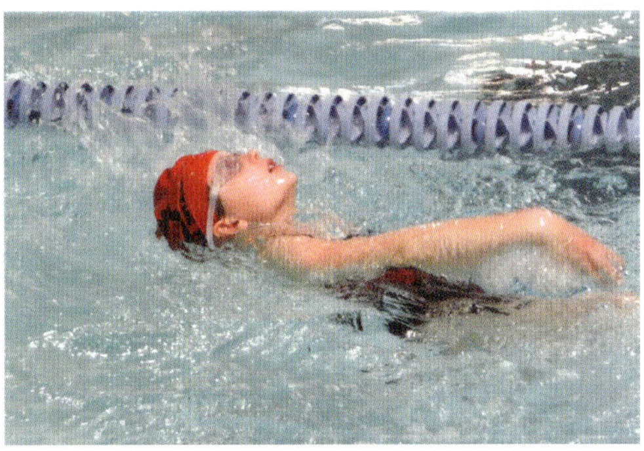

A swimmer focuses on the ceiling while doing the backstroke.

Approaching the wall has the problem that the swimmer cannot see where he or she is going. Most competitive swimmers know how many strokes they need for a lane, or at least how many strokes after the signal flags or the change in color of the separating lines. Turning the head is also possible, but slows the swimmer down.

Prior to September 1992 swimmers had to touch the wall on their back before initiating the turn or rolling off their back in order to turn. After September 1992 when approaching the wall, the swimmer is allowed to turn to his or her breast and make one push/pull phase with one arm or simultaneous double arm pull. Next, the swimmer makes half a tumble turn forward, resting the feet against the wall. The arms are in the forward position at this time, and the swimmer pushes their body off the wall. Similar to the start, the swimmer can remain up to 15 m under water, with most swimmers using a butterfly kick for speed. This rule change allowed for faster turns.

For the finish, the swimmer must touch the wall while lying on his back, less than 90 degrees out of the horizontal, and must not be completely submerged.

Reasons to Flip to Backstroke

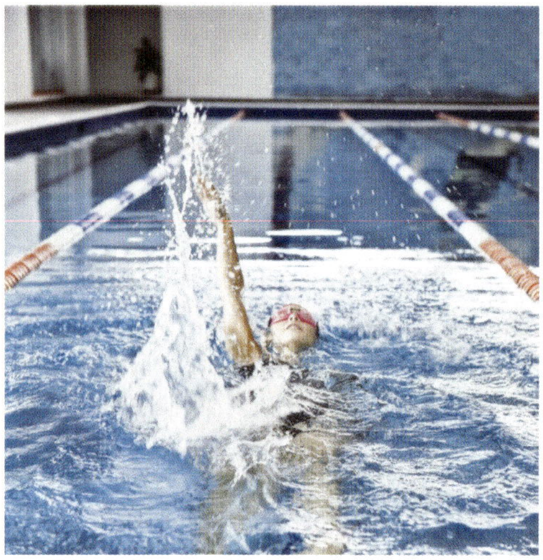

1. Improves your posture: Backstroke is a great exercise to reverse the effects of time spent on the computer. Unlike most of our daily activities — or even other swimming strokes — backstroke helps open up chest muscles. Backstroke also strengthens the upper back and lats, pulling your shoulders back, which helps create better posture.

2. Tightens your core: The key to backstroke is balance. Although all swim strokes strengthen the abs, the rhythm of backstroke engages your entire core through a slight hip rotation. In addition, the undulating movement from the kicks off of each wall, activates both your lower back and core.

3. Can be used as cross-training for runners: If you're a runner, swimming is a low-impact way to cross train between runs. Backstroke kicks engage the muscles in your legs and glutes for a complete lower-body workout; further challenged by the resistance of the water.

4. Complements freestyle: As with every exercise routine, balance is key. Freestyle is often favored by many swimmers and is the first stroke taught to beginners. Mix up your work-outs and improve your freestyle by incorporating a few laps of backstroke into your regime. Freestyle and backstroke are perfect complements to each other, working opposite muscle groups. Consider alternating strokes between laps or using backstroke to cool down with.

5. Will improve your weight-room workout: When you're not rocking it out in the weight room, use backstroke as a way to straighten your arms and shoulders. Once your fingers enter the water to begin your catch, your biceps must bend against the resistance of the water to finish each stroke. Although your biceps and lats are in the greatest demand during the catch, your triceps and lats will benefit as well.

Sidestroke

The sidestroke is a swim stroke swum on the sides. It is not used in competitions and therefore less known nowadays. Because it is swum on the side and uses asymmetrical movements of the limbs, it can look peculiar the first time you see it. Nevertheless it can add some variety to your swim sessions.

Every recreational and professional swimmer can learn swim the sidestroke because it is useful in so many ways:

- The stroke is often needed when rescuing someone from the water. If you are pulling someone from the water, you will need to swim on your side so you can pull them without losing speed, and without drowning yourself along with them.
- You can go faster with the sidestroke than the breaststroke, which is originally why this stroke was created. You do not have the pressure of your body against the water to hold you back, so you go faster with each kick when performing this stroke.
- Breathing technique is simple and easy to learn with this stroke. In fact, many people find the entire stroke to be rather simple to learn.
- It allows your face and one ear to remain out of the water, so it is great for swimmers who do not want to keep their face down in the water.
- You work a lot of muscles with the sidestroke, but it is still incredibly relaxing. You get some fitness benefits while relaxing.

You can perform the sidestroke quickly, or in a more relaxing manner. The stroke is performed entirely on your side, and your body is propelled forward by a combination of a scissor style kick and the force of your lead arm. Your lead arm is the arm under the water, beneath your body when you are turned on your side.

Performing the Sidestroke

Stand in the water, and then turn your body to the side with one arm under the water, and the other on top. Your top arm should be down by your thigh, while your lead arm extends out in front of your body in the water.

Push off with your legs, keeping them close together. Your leg motion will be like scissors, with one leg going forward while the other goes back, and then switching. While your legs are kicking, your lead arm should push down into the water, drawing toward the body and then back out. Keep the hand of your lead arm turned with the palm facing out in front of your body and a little downward.

Chapter 5

Weight Training

Weight training is a form of strength training that involves the development of strength and size of the skeletal muscles, using dumbbells, weighted bars and weight stacks. A weight training regime is a significant aspect of physical education. This chapter discusses in detail the relevant weight training exercises, such as squats, leg presses, biceps training, triceps training, etc.

Weight training is a type of strength training that uses weights for resistance. Weight training provides a stress to the muscles that causes them to adapt and get stronger, similar to the way aerobic conditioning strengthens your heart.

Weight training can be performed with free weights, such as barbells and dumbbells, or by using weight machines. You can also increase your strength through other types of resistance exercises, such as by using your body weight or resistance bands.

Most of us know that cardio is important for getting fit and losing some weight, but what you may not know is just how important weight training is when it comes to getting lean and burning fat.

A session of weight training doesn't always burn as many calories in one sitting as cardio and, of course, cardio is important for weight loss. However, if you really want to change your body and make a difference, you need to lift weights.

Weight training involves using some type of resistance to do a variety of exercises designed to challenge all your muscle groups, including your chest, back, shoulder, biceps, triceps, core, and lower body.

The idea is that, when you use more resistance than your body normally handles, your muscles get stronger, along with your bones and connective tissue, all while building lean muscle tissue.

That lean muscle tissue is more metabolically active than fat, which means you burn more calories all day long, even when you're not exercising.

Weight training doesn't mean you have to use things like dumbbells or machines, although those work. Anything that provides resistance can do the job—resistance bands, barbells, a heavy backpack, or, if you're a beginner, your own body weight might be enough to get you started.

Weight Training Versus Other Types of Exercise

Strength training is an inclusive term that describes all exercises devoted toward increasing physical strength. Weight training is a type of strength training that uses weights, Eccentric Training or muscular resistance to increase strength. Endurance training is associated with aerobic exercise while flexibility training is associated with stretching exercise like yoga or pilates. *Weight training* is often used as a synonym for strength training, but is actually a specific type within the more inclusive category. Contrary to popular belief, weight training can be beneficial for both men and women.

Comparison to other Types of Strength Training

The benefits of weight training overall are comparable to most other types of strength training: increased muscle, tendon and ligament strength, bone density, flexibility, tone, metabolic rate, and postural support. This type of training will also help prevent injury for athletes. There are benefits and limitations to weight training as compared to other types of strength training.

Weight Training Versus Isometric Training

Isometric exercise provides a maximum amount of resistance based on the force output of the muscle, or muscles pitted against one another. This maximum force maximally strengthens the muscles over all of the joint angles at which the isometric exercise occurs. By comparison, weight training also strengthens the muscle throughout the range of motion the joint is trained in, but only maximally at one angle, causing a lesser increase in physical strength at other angles from the initial through terminating joint angle as compared with isometric exercise. In addition, the risk of injury from weights used in weight training is greater than with isometric exercise (no weights), and the risk of asymmetric training is also greater than with isometric exercise of identical opposing muscles.

Weight Training and Bodybuilding

Although weight training is similar to bodybuilding, they have different objectives. Bodybuilders use weight training to develop their muscles for size, shape, and symmetry regardless of any increase in strength for competition in bodybuilding contests; they train to maximize their muscular size and develop extremely low levels of body fat. In contrast, many weight trainers train to improve their strength and anaerobic endurance while not giving special attention to reducing body fat far below normal.

The bodybuilding community has been the source of many weight training principles, techniques, vocabulary, and customs. Weight training does allow tremendous flexibility in exercises and weights which can allow bodybuilders to target specific muscles and muscle groups, as well as attain specific goals. Not all bodybuilding is undertaken to compete in bodybuilding contests and, in fact, the vast majority of bodybuilders never compete, but bodybuild for their own personal reasons.

Complex Training

In complex training, weight training is typically combined with plyometric exercises in an alternating sequence. Ideally, the weight lifting exercise and the plyometric exercise should move through similar ranges of movement i.e. a back squat at 85-95% 1RM followed by a vertical jump. An advantage of this form of training is that it allows the intense activation of the nervous system and increased muscle fibre recruitment from the weight lifting exercise to be utilized in the subsequent plyometric exercise; thereby improving the power with which it can be performed. Over a period of training, this may enhance the athlete's ability to apply power.

Ballistic Training

Ballistic training incorporates weight training in such a way that the acceleration phase of the movement is maximized and the deceleration phase minimized; thereby increasing the power of the movement overall. For example, throwing a weight or jumping whilst holding a weight. This can be contrasted with a standard weight lifting exercise where there is a distinct deceleration phase at the end of the repetition which stops the weight from moving.

Contrast Loading

Contrast loading is the alternation of heavy and light loads. Considered as sets, the heavy load is performed at about 85-95% 1 repetition max; the light load should be considerably lighter at about 30-60% 1RM. Both sets should be performed fast with the lighter set being performed as fast as possible. The joints should not be locked as this inhibits muscle fibre recruitment and reduces the speed at which the exercise can be performed. The lighter set may be a loaded plyometric exercise such as loaded squat jumps or jumps with a trap bar.

Similarly to complex training, contrast loading relies upon the enhanced activation of the nervous system and increased muscle fibre recruitment from the heavy set, to allow the lighter set to be performed more powerfully. Such a physiological effect is commonly referred to as post-activation potentiation, or the PAP effect. Contrast loading can effectively demonstrate the PAP effect: if a light weight is lifted, and then a heavy weight is lifted, and then the same light weight is lifted again, then the light weight will feel lighter the second time it has been lifted. This is due to the enhanced PAP effect which occurs as a result of the heavy lift being utilised in the subsequent lighter lift; thus making the weight feel lighter and allowing the lift to be performed more powerfully.

Safety

Weight training is a safe form of exercise when the movements are controlled and carefully defined. However, as with any form of exercise, improper execution and the failure to take appropriate precautions can result in injury.

Maintaining Proper Form

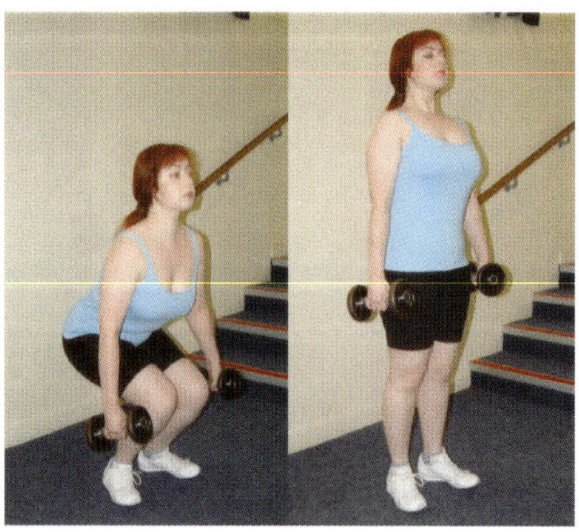

A dumbbell half-squat.

Maintaining proper form is one of the many steps in order to perfectly perform a certain technique. Correct form in weight training improves strength, muscle tone, and maintaining a healthy weight. Proper form will prevent any strains or fractures. When the exercise becomes difficult towards the end of a set, there is a temptation to cheat, i.e., to use poor form to recruit other muscle groups to assist the effort. Avoid heavy weight and keep the number of repetitions to a minimum. This may shift the effort to weaker muscles that cannot handle the weight. For example, the *squat* and the *deadlift* are used to exercise the largest muscles in the body—the leg and buttock muscles—so they require substantial weight. Beginners are tempted to round their back while performing these exercises. The relaxation of the spinal erectors which allows the lower back to round can cause shearing in the vertebrae of the lumbar spine, potentially damaging the spinal discs.

Stretching and Warm-up

Weight trainers commonly spend 5 to 20 minutes warming up their muscles before starting a workout. It is common to stretch the entire body to increase overall flexibility; however, many people stretch just the area being worked that day. The main reason for warming up is injury prevention. Warming up increases blood flow and flexibility, which lessens the chance of a muscle pull or joint pain.

Warm up sets are also important. For example, the same lifter working on his chest would also be advised to complete at least two warm up sets prior to hitting his "core tonnage." Core tonnage refers to the heavier lifts that actually strain your muscles. For example, if the lifter's main sets were at 205 lbs, 225 lbs and 235 lbs on the bench, then a warmup of 5 reps of 135 and 5 reps of 185 would be advisable. Some lifters will warm up with a 50/50 set for example 50% of the target weight for 50% of the target repetitions. When properly warmed up the lifter will then have more strength and stamina since the blood has begun to flow to the muscle groups.

Breathing

In weight training, as with most forms of exercise, there is a tendency for the breathing pattern to deepen. This helps to meet increased oxygen requirements. Holding the breath or breathing shallowly is avoided because it may lead to a lack of oxygen, passing out, or an excessive build up of blood pressure. Generally, the recommended breathing technique is to inhale when lowering the weight (the eccentric portion) and exhale when lifting the weight (the concentric portion). However, the reverse, inhaling when lifting and exhaling when lowering, may also be recommended. Some researchers state that there is little difference between the two techniques in terms of their influence on heart rate and blood pressure. It may also be recommended that a weight lifter simply breathes in a manner which feels appropriate.

Deep breathing may be specifically recommended for the lifting of heavy weights because it helps to generate intra-abdominal pressure which can help to strengthen the posture of the lifter, and especially their core.

In particular situations, a coach may advise performing the valsalva maneuver during exercises which place a load on the spine, since the risk of a stroke by aneurysm is astronomically lower than the risk of an orthopedic injury caused by inadequate rigidity of the torso. Stuart McGill adds that the mechanism of building "high levels of intra-abdominal pressure (IAP) produced by breath holding using the Valsava maneuver", to "ensure spine stiffness and stability during these extraordinary demands", "should be considered only for extreme weight-lifting challenges — not for rehabilitation exercise".

Hydration

As with other sports, weight trainers should avoid dehydration throughout the workout by drinking sufficient water. This is particularly true in hot environments, or for those older than 65.

Some athletic trainers advise athletes to drink about 7 imperial fluid ounces (200 mL) every 15 minutes while exercising, and about 80 imperial fluid ounces (2.3 L) throughout the day.

However, a much more accurate determination of how much fluid is necessary can be made by performing appropriate weight measurements before and after a typical exercise session, to determine how much fluid is lost during the workout. The greatest source of fluid loss during exercise is through perspiration, but as long as your fluid intake is roughly equivalent to your rate of perspiration, hydration levels will be maintained.

Under most circumstances, sports drinks do not offer a physiological benefit over water during weight training. However, high-intensity exercise for a continuous duration of at least one hour may require the replenishment of electrolytes which a sports drink may provide. Some may maintain that energy drinks, such as Red Bull that contain caffeine, improve performance in weight training and other physical exercise, but in fact, these energy drinks can cause dehydration, tremors, heat stroke, and heart attack when consumed in excess.'Sports drinks' that contain simple carbohydrates & water do not cause ill effects, but are most likely unnecessary for the average trainee. More recently, people have been taking pre-workout before working out to increase performance. The main ingredients in these pre-workouts are: beta-alanine, creatine, BCAAs (branched chain amino acids) and caffeine.

Insufficient hydration may cause lethargy, soreness or muscle cramps. The urine of well-hydrated persons should be nearly colorless, while an intense yellow color is normally a sign of insufficient hydration.

Avoiding Pain

An exercise should be halted if marked or sudden pain is felt, to prevent further injury. However, not all discomfort indicates injury. Weight training exercises are brief but very intense, and many people are unaccustomed to this level of effort. The expression "no pain, no gain" refers to working through the discomfort expected from such vigorous effort, rather than to willfully ignore extreme pain, which may indicate serious soft tissue injuries. The focus must be proper form, not the amount of weight lifted.

Discomfort can arise from other factors. Individuals who perform large numbers of repetitions, sets, and exercises for each muscle group may experience a burning sensation in their muscles. These individuals may also experience a swelling sensation in their muscles from increased blood flow (the "pump"). True muscle fatigue is experienced as a marked and uncontrollable loss of strength in a muscle, arising from the nervous system (motor unit) rather than from the muscle fibers themselves. Extreme neural fatigue can be experienced as temporary muscle failure. Some weight training programs, such as Metabolic Resistance Training, actively seek temporary muscle failure; evidence to support this type of training is mixed at best. Irrespective of their program, however, most athletes engaged in high-intensity weight training will experience muscle failure during their regimens.

Beginners are advised to build up slowly to a weight training program. Untrained individuals may have some muscles that are comparatively stronger than others. An injury can result if, in a particular exercise, the primary muscle is stronger than its stabilising muscles. Building up slowly allows muscles time to develop appropriate strengths relative to each other. This can also help to minimize delayed onset muscle soreness. A sudden start to an intense program can cause significant muscular soreness. Unexercised muscles contain cross-linkages that are torn during intense exercise. A regimen of flexibility exercises should be implemented before weight training begins, to help avoid soft tissue pain and injuries.

Other Precautions

Anyone beginning an intensive physical training program is typically advised to consult a physician, because of possible undetected heart or other conditions for which such activity is contraindicated.

Exercises like the bench press or the squat in which a failed lift can potentially result in the lifter becoming trapped under the weight are normally performed inside a power rack or in the presence of one or more spotters, who can safely re-rack the barbell if the weight trainer is unable to do so.

Equipment

Weight training usually requires different types of equipment, most commonly dumbbells, barbells, weight plates, and weight machines. Various combinations of specific exercises, machines, dumbbells, and barbells allow trainees to exercise body parts in numerous ways.

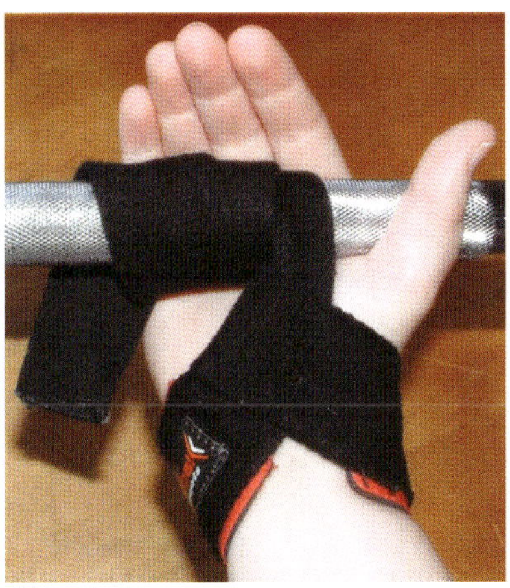

A lifting strap.

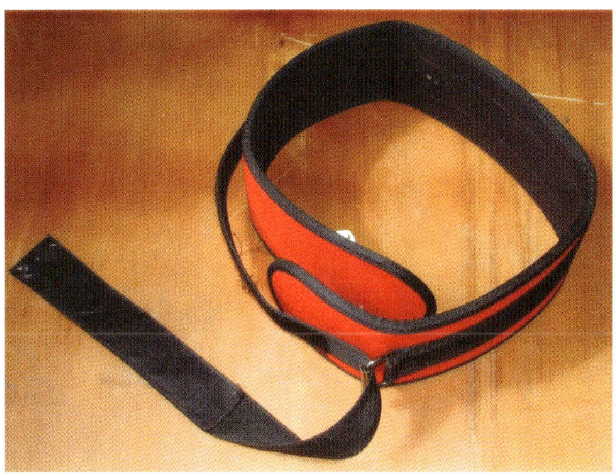

A lifting belt.

Other types of equipment include:

- Lifting straps, which allow more weight to be lifted by transferring the load to the wrists and avoiding limitations in forearm muscles and grip strength
- Weightlifting belts, which are meant to brace the core through intra-abdominal pressure. Controversy exists regarding the safety of these devices and their proper use is often misunderstood
- Weighted clothing, bags of sand, lead shot, or other materials that are strapped to wrists, ankles, torso or other body parts to increase the amount of work required by muscles
- Gloves can improve grip, prevent the formation of calluses on the hands, relieve pressure on the wrists, and provide support
- Chalk ($MgCO_3$), which dries out sweaty hands, improving grip
- Wrist and knee wraps
- Shoes, which have a flat, rigid sole to provide a sturdy base of support, and may feature a raised heel of varying height (usually 0.5" or 0.75") to accommodate a lifter's biomechanics for more efficient squats, deadlifts, overhead presses, and Olympic lifts.

Types of Exercises

Isotonic and Plyometric Exercises

These terms combine the prefix *iso-* (meaning "same") with *tonic* ("strength") and *plio-* ("more") with *metric* ("distance"). In "isotonic" exercises the force applied to the muscle does not change (while the length of the muscle decreases or increases) while in "plyometric" exercises the length of the muscle stretches and contracts rapidly to increase the power output of a muscle.

Weight training is primarily an isotonic form of exercise, as the force produced by the muscle to push or pull weighted objects should not change (though in practice the force produced does decrease as muscles fatigue). Any object can be used for weight training, but dumbbells, barbells, and other specialised equipment are normally used because they can be adjusted to specific weights and are easily gripped. Many exercises are not strictly isotonic because the force on the muscle varies as the joint moves through its range of motion. Movements can become easier or harder depending on the angle of muscular force relative to gravity; for example, a standard biceps curl becomes easier as the hand approaches the shoulder as more of the load is taken by the structure of the elbow. Originating from Nautilus, Inc., some machines use a logarithmic-spiral cam to keep resistance constant irrespective of the joint angle.

Plyometrics exploit the stretch-shortening cycle of muscles to enhance the myotatic (stretch) reflex. This involves rapid alternation of lengthening and shortening of muscle fibers against resistance. The resistance involved is often a weighted object such as a medicine ball or sandbag, but can also be the body itself as in jumping exercises or the body with a weight vest that allows movement with resistance. Plyometrics is used to develop explosive speed, and focuses on maximal power instead of maximal strength by compressing the force of muscular contraction into as short a period as possible, and may be used to improve the effectiveness of a boxer's punch, or to increase the vertical jumping ability of a basketball player. Care must be taken when performing plyometric exercises because they inflict greater stress upon the involved joints and tendons than other forms of exercise.

Isolation Exercises Versus Compound Exercises

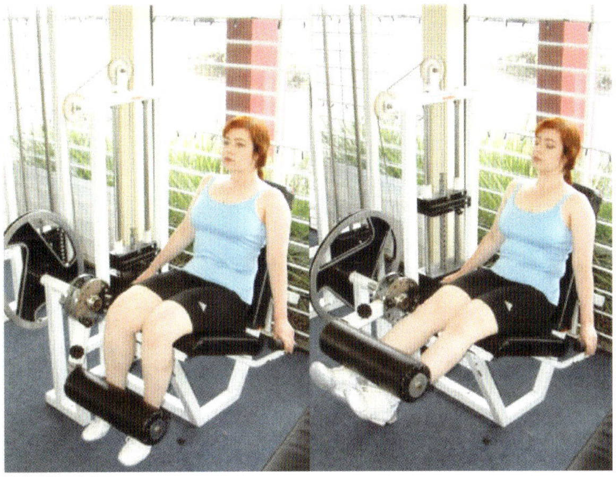

The *leg extension* is an isolation exercise.

An isolation exercise is one where the movement is restricted to one joint only. For example, the *leg extension* is an isolation exercise for the quadriceps. Specialized types of equipment are used to ensure that other muscle groups are only minimally involved—they just help the individual maintain a stable posture—and movement occurs only around the knee joint. Most isolation exercises involve machines rather than dumbbells and barbells (free weights), though free weights can be used when combined with special positions and joint bracing.

Compound exercises work several muscle groups at once, and include movement around two or more joints. For example, in the *leg press*, movement occurs around the hip, knee and ankle joints. This exercise is primarily used to develop the quadriceps, but it also involves the hamstrings, glutes and calves. Compound exercises are generally similar to the ways that people naturally push, pull and lift objects, whereas isolation exercises often feel a little unnatural.

Each type of exercise has its uses. Compound exercises build the basic strength that is needed to perform everyday pushing, pulling and lifting activities. Isolation exercises are useful for "rounding out" a routine, by directly exercising muscle groups that cannot be fully exercised in the compound exercises.

The type of exercise performed also depends on the individual's goals. Those who seek to increase their performance in sports would focus mostly on compound exercises, with isolation exercises being used to strengthen just those muscles that are holding the athlete back. Similarly, a powerlifter would focus on the specific compound exercises that are performed at powerlifting competitions. However, those who seek to improve the look of their body without necessarily maximizing their strength gains (including bodybuilders) would put more of an emphasis on isolation exercises. Both types of athletes, however, generally make use of both compound and isolation exercises.

Free Weights Versus Weight Machines

Free weights include dumbbells, barbells, medicine balls, sandbells, and kettlebells. Unlike weight machines, they do not constrain users to specific, fixed movements, and therefore require more effort from the individual's stabilizer muscles. It is often argued that free weight exercises are superior for precisely this reason. For example, they are recommended for golf players, since golf is a unilateral exercise that can break body balances, requiring exercises to keep the balance in muscles.

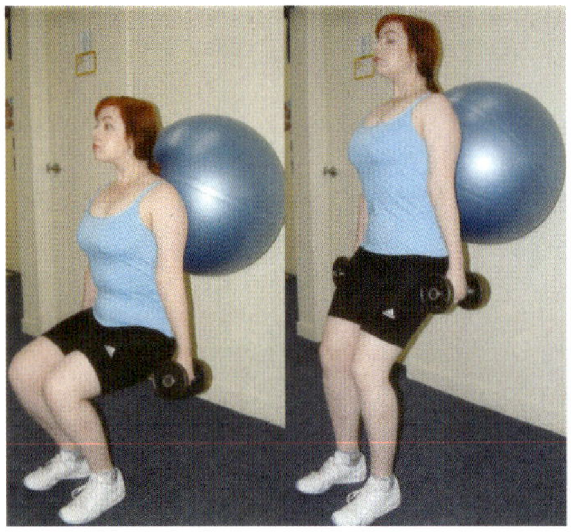

Exercise balls allow a wider range of free weight exercises to be performed. They are also known as Swiss balls, stability balls, fitness balls, gym balls, sports balls, therapy balls or body balls. They are sometimes confused with medicine balls.

Some free weight exercises can be performed while sitting or lying on an exercise ball.

There are a number of weight machines that are commonly found in neighborhood gyms. The Smith machine is a barbell that is constrained to vertical movement. The cable machine consists of two weight stacks separated by 2.5 metres, with cables running through adjustable pulleys (that can be fixed at any height) to various types of handles. There are also exercise-specific weight machines such as the leg press. A multigym includes a variety of exercise-specific mechanisms in one apparatus.

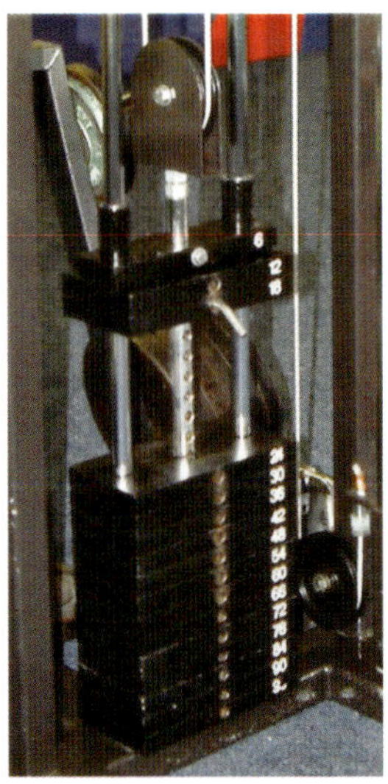

The weight stack from a cable machine.

One limitation of many free weight exercises and exercise machines is that the muscle is working maximally against gravity during only a small portion of the lift. Some exercise-specific machines feature an oval cam (first introduced by Nautilus) which varies the resistance, so that the resistance, and the muscle force required, remains constant throughout the full range of motion of the exercise.

Push-pull Workout

A push–pull workout is a method of arranging a weight training routine so that exercises alternate between push motions and pull motions. A push–pull superset is two complementary segments (one pull/one push) done back-to-back. An example is bench press (push) / bent-over row (pull). Another push–pull technique is to arrange workout routines so that one day involves only push (usually chest, shoulders and triceps) exercises, and an alternate day only pull (usually back and biceps) exercises so the body can get adequate rest.

Health Benefits

Benefits of weight training include increased strength, muscle mass, endurance, bone and bone mineral density, insulin sensitivity, GLUT 4 density, HDL cholesterol, improved cardiovascular health and appearance, and decreased body fat, blood pressure, LDL cholesterol and triglycerides.

The body's basal metabolic rate increases with increases in muscle mass, which promotes long-term fat loss and helps dieters avoid yo-yo dieting. Moreover, intense workouts elevate metabolism for several hours following the workout, which also promotes fat loss.

Weight training also provides functional benefits. Stronger muscles improve posture, provide better support for joints, and reduce the risk of injury from everyday activities. Older people who take up weight training can prevent some of the loss of muscle tissue that normally accompanies aging—and even regain some functional strength—and by doing so, become less frail. They may be able to avoid some types of physical disability. Weight-bearing exercise also helps to prevent osteoporosis. The benefits of weight training for older people have been confirmed by studies of people who began engaging in it even in their eighties and nineties.

For many people in rehabilitation or with an acquired disability, such as following stroke or orthopaedic surgery, strength training for weak muscles is a key factor to optimise recovery. For people with such a health condition, their strength training is likely to need to be designed by an appropriate health professional, such as a physiotherapist.

Stronger muscles improve performance in a variety of sports. Sport-specific training routines are used by many competitors. These often specify that the speed of muscle contraction during weight training should be the same as that of the particular sport. Sport-specific training routines also often include variations to both free weight and machine movements that may not be common for traditional weightlifting.

Though weight training can stimulate the cardiovascular system, many exercise physiologists, based on their observation of maximal oxygen uptake, argue that aerobics training is a better cardiovascular stimulus. Central catheter monitoring during resistance training reveals increased cardiac output, suggesting that strength training shows potential for cardiovascular exercise.

However, a 2007 meta-analysis found that, though aerobic training is an effective therapy for heart failure patients, combined aerobic and strength training is ineffective; "the favorable antiremodeling role of aerobic exercise was not confirmed when this mode of exercise was combined with strength training".

One side-effect of any intense exercise is increased levels of dopamine, serotonin and norepinephrine, which can help to improve mood and counter feelings of depression.

Weight training has also been shown to benefit dieters as it inhibits lean body mass loss (as opposed to fat loss) when under a caloric deficit. Weight training also strengthens bones, helping to prevent bone loss and osteoporosis. By increasing muscular strength and improving balance, weight training can also reduce falls by elderly persons. Weight training is also attracting attention for the benefits it can have on the brain, and in older adults, a 2017 meta analysis found that it was effective in improving cognitive performance.

Free Weights

A free weight exercise is any exercise where the resistance is provided by a barbell, dumbbells, or any other *free* moving object. Some common examples include any type of barbell or dumbbell press, row, curl, extension, or deadlift.

Basically, if you're moving some sort of weight (like a barbell or dumbbell) from point A to point B, and that weight isn't supported by or attached to anything other than you, it's most likely a free weight exercise.

PROS

- Completely natural movement. Allows you to move through a range of motion that is completely natural for your specific body. Nothing is restricted or put into any sort of fixed position that may not be perfect for you body.
- Uses additional muscles. Since you are in full control of the weight and stabilizing the entire movement itself, you are therefore recruiting the use of various stabilizer muscles that tend to go unused with machines.
- Extremely functional. Free weight exercises allow you to mimic actual movements that you actually do in real life, and in the exact manner you'd actually do them.
- Ideal for home use. If you happen to do your weight training at home, a barbell (or dumbbells), some weight and a bench is all you need to be able to perform dozens of different exercises in your house.

CONS

- Usually harder to learn at first. Especially when compared to machines (and to a lesser extent, body weight exercises), it's usually a little harder to learn proper technique as a beginner.
- Higher *potential* risk of injury. There is a risk of injury with every type of exercise, but the potential may be a little bit higher with free weights than others.

Types of Free Weight

1. Dumbbells

The most popular type of free weight, dumbbells are a great addition to your home gym and the first port of call for many gym newbies.

"Dumbbells can be extremely effective because you have to use each side of your body individually," This helps ensure you don't have any body parts that lag behind, because your weaker side can't rely on your stronger side to do the rep.

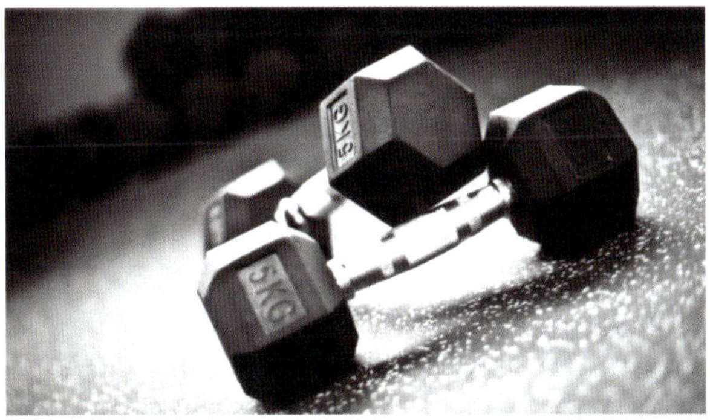

"The uneven and unstable nature of using dumbbells will also ensure your core gets a good workout as it'll be fighting to keep you stable throughout the movement.

The primary downside of dumbbells is that you can't stack huge amounts of weight on them.

"If you want to lift as heavy as possible and focus on compound moves like squats and deadlifts, a barbell will be more effective,"

2. Kettlebells

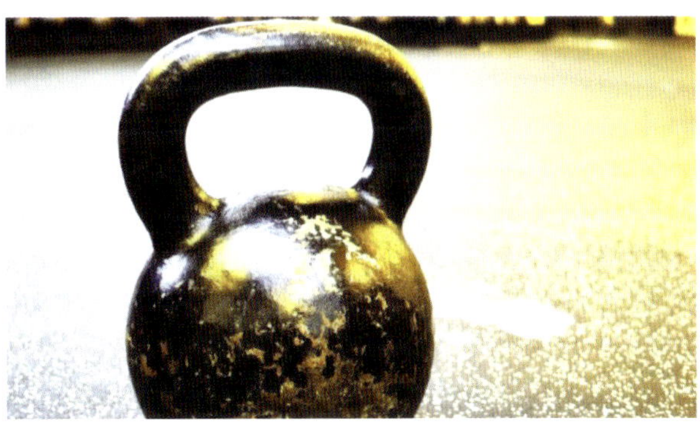

If you're a fan of functional training, you should be using kettlebells, because their shape and the way you hold them allows you to mimic natural movements more easily than with dumbbells.

"Exercises like kettlebell swings help you to build up your glute strength while your body swings and your hips thrust in a natural pattern.

However, as with dumbbells, there's a limit to how heavy you can go with kettlebells.

3. Barbells and Plates

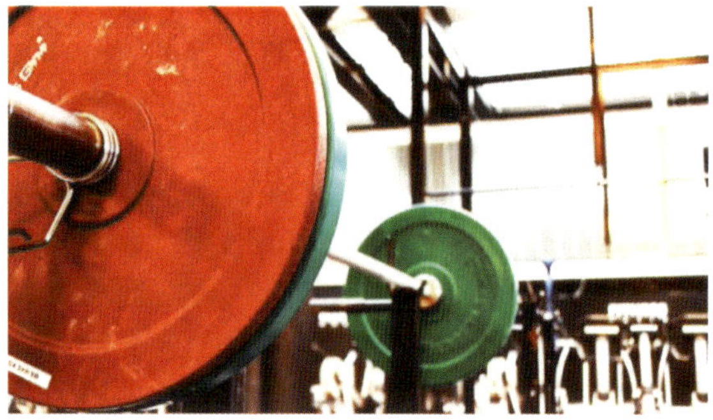

"If you're looking to build strength and size, you'll want to lift as heavy a weight as possible – making sure you're doing so with perfect form, This is where barbells and plates come into their own.

"You do barbell exercises using both sides of your body, which means you're able to lift a lot more weight. It's also far more stable and balanced than using dumbbells, but you'll still have to use your core because it's less stable than using machines."

Before you head straight for the barbell, remember there are downsides too. Using them can be tough on your wrists and you can't move as freely as with dumbbells or kettlebells.

"You're a little limited in your range of movement when using a barbell, There are certain exercises like the bench press where you're forced to stop because of the bar, rather than where your flexibility would allow you to move."

4. EZ-bar

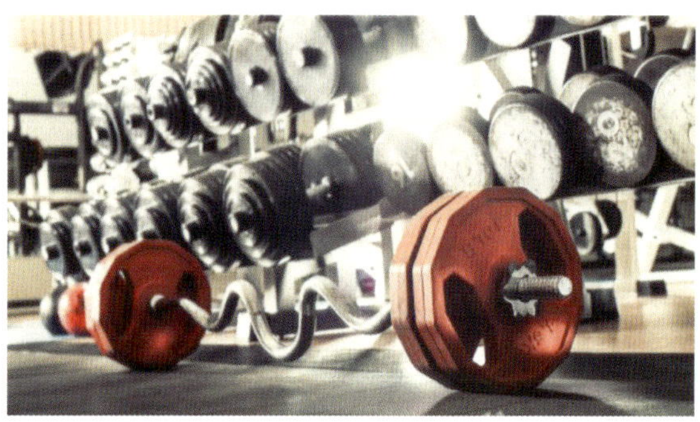

This bar differs from the standard straight bar by bending in a slight zig-zag pattern in the middle, which makes certain exercises a little easier on your wrists.

"EZ-bars are great for allowing you to get the leverage to go heavy – especially on biceps and triceps exercises – without straining your wrists and forcing them into unnatural positions,"

The EZ-bar shares some disadvantages with the standard barbell, the main one being that it can mask weaknesses in your body.

"As with the barbell, the EZ-bar means your weaker side can get a slightly easier ride because the stronger side can do most the work in the rep."

5. Sandbags/Sandbells

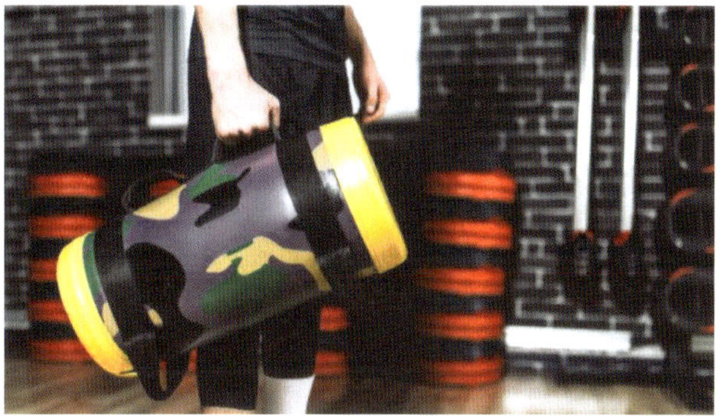

Sand-filled weights can be just as heavy as dumbbells and kettlebells, but they're not as hard, so you can throw them around and slam them down without wrecking floors and walls.

"In a similar way to kettlebells, sandbags allow you to build functional strength and replicate more natural movements." "The design of the bags allows you to move as your body wants to, as opposed to being restricted to where a solid bar dictates."

Sandbags and bells can be cumbersome, however, and they're not the best for lifting massive weight.

"You won't be able to go as heavy as possible with these – they're more for building stamina."

Benefits of Using Free Weights

When you use free weights you get more bang for your buck. There are loads of exercises that one can do with free weights. And these can be done at home or at the gym than one can do with the big expensive machines.

While doing free weights there is no range of motion inhibitors like with most exercise machines. You can adjust each exercise according to your body. Another great benefit with free weight is that you can really enhance your motor skills. When using free weights their are more action on your muscles to stabilize and balance your body and its weight thereby giving you a more complete workout.

Ideally if you are serious and you want get strong the you need to train on free weights.

Firstly, you will need advice to help you get the right workout program design. Hiring a trainer or researching the best exercises for you must come first. It is also extremely important to use proper form. Thus, hiring a trainer will get you started right.

Secondly, the chances of getting injured is higher while using free weights. If you don't lift it right and do the exercises in the right manner, free weights can hurt you faster than it will make you fit.

Thirdly, You will need a lifting partner if you plan on pumping heavy iron. Get a partner or a trainer to help check your form. It is very easy to get sloppy, even when you know what your doing. For example, don't try a heavy weight in the squat or bench press without a "spotter". Make sure that you can control the weight and do the exercise correctly and in the right position.

Isometric Exercise

Isometric exercises are contractions of a particular muscle or group of muscles. During isometric exercises, the muscle doesn't noticeably change length and the affected joint doesn't move. Isometric exercises help maintain strength. They can also build strength, but not effectively.

Because isometric exercises are done in one position without movement, they'll improve strength in only one particular position. You'd have to do various isometric exercises through your limb's whole range of motion to improve muscle strength across the range. In addition, since isometric exercises are done in a static position, they won't help improve speed or athletic performance. They can be useful, however, in enhancing stabilization — maintaining the position of the affected area — since muscles often contract isometrically to aid in stabilization.

Isometric Exercises And Their Benefits

1. Plank

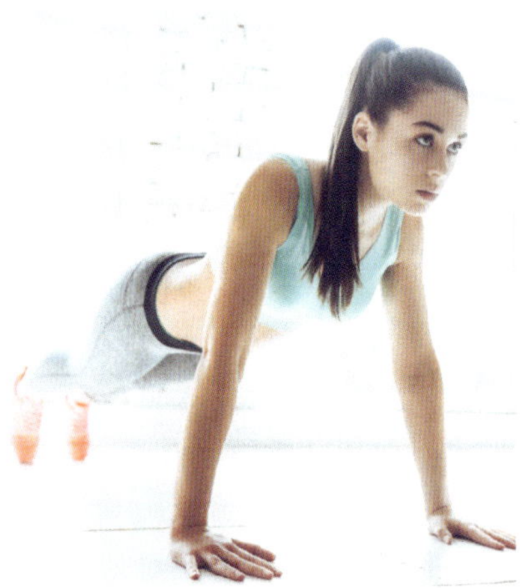

Target

Transversus abdominis muscle, gluteus minimus muscles, gluteus medius, adductor muscles of the hip, and obliques.

Starting Position

Get into the push-up position with your arms straight, abs tight, belly button sucked in, and body straight.

Steps To Do

1. Hold this pose for 10-15 seconds.
2. Slowly get back to the starting position and repeat.
3. Try increasing the holding time gradually.

Precaution

Do not stress too much right in the beginning. Build your strength gradually.

2. Forearm Plank

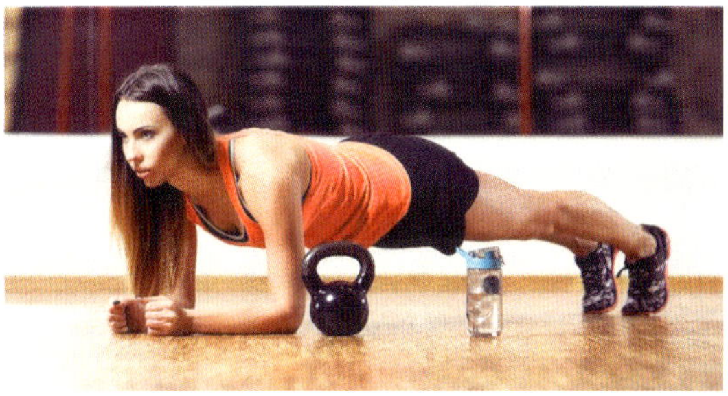

Target

Transversus abdominis muscle, gluteus minimus muscles, gluteus medius, adductor muscles of the hip, and obliques.

Starting Position

Start in the plank position with your body straight and abs tight.

Steps To Do

1. Bend your arms. Lower your body, concentrating the weight on your forearms.
2. Hold the pose for 10 seconds. Try to increase the holding time gradually.
3. Slowly get back to the starting position and repeat.

Repetitions

5 reps to complete 1 set.

Precaution

Do not point your elbows outward or inward. Place them close your body.

3. Side Plank

Target

Transversus abdominis, rectus abdominis, obliques, quadratus lumborum. gluteus medius, gluteus minimus, and adductors.

Starting Position

Get into the plank position with all the muscles tensed.

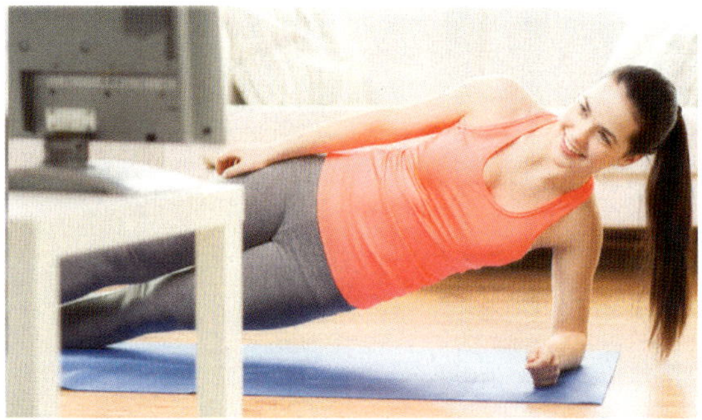

Steps To Do

1. Shift your weight slowly to your right side and balance with one hand and foot on the ground.
2. Extend your left hand straight into the air and put your left foot over the right one.
3. Hold the pose for 10 seconds. Repeat on the other side.
4. Slowly get back to the starting position and repeat.

Repetitions

5 reps to complete 1 set.

Precaution

If extending your hand makes you unstable, keep your hand on your waist as you do the plank.

4. Isometric Push-up

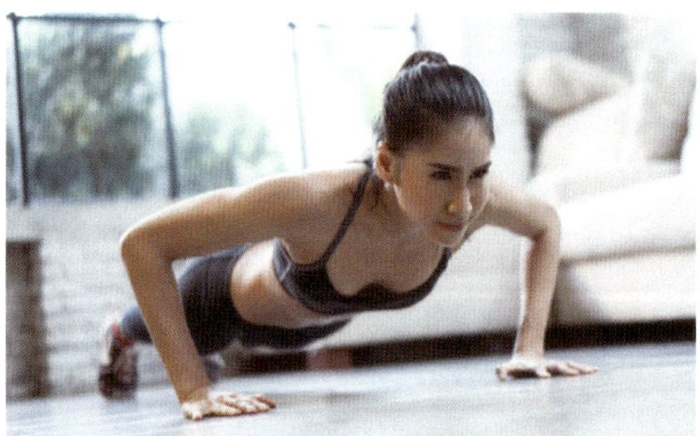

Target

Abs, middle and lower back, triceps, and chest.

Starting Position

To begin with, one must assume the normal push-up position and balance the body on the knees and palms.

Steps To Do

Slowly raise the body upwards, holding it for one second before coming down.

This may sound easy, but it might be challenging to hold the position when the weight of the entire body falls on the palms and the knees.

Repetitions

10 reps to complete 1 set.

Precaution

Do not stress too much right in the beginning. Build your strength gradually.

5. Isometric Low Plank

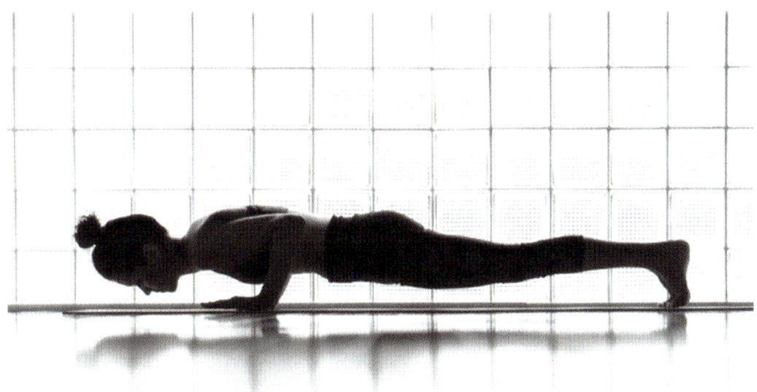

The isometric low plank is a combination of the plank and the push-up. This is a great exercise for those who want to build core strength and get toned arms, a flat tummy, and well-shaped shoulders.

Target

Abs, middle and lower back, biceps, triceps, and glutes.

Starting Position

Assume the push-up position.

Steps To Do

1. Lower your body. Bend your elbows, keep your head up, and chin straight.
2. Slowly push your upper body up as you straighten your elbows and support your body weight with your arms, shoulders, and palms.
3. Hold it for 5 seconds.
4. Lower your body and hold for 5 seconds.

Repetitions

5 reps to complete 1 set.

Precaution

Make sure your body is well supported by your toes and your elbows.

Isometric Exercises For The Shoulders

6. Hanging

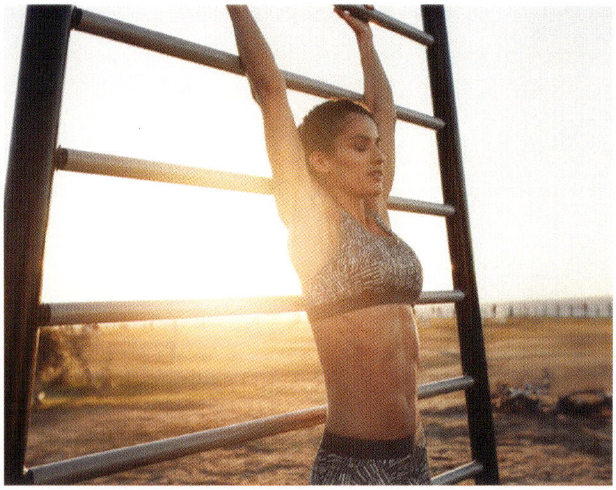

Target

Shoulders, lats, upper abs, obliques, biceps, and triceps.

Starting Position

Grab a pull-up bar or any other bar type surface from which you can properly hang.

Steps To Do

1. Hold the bar with your hand and hang.
2. Hang there for 10-15 seconds and then come down.

Repetitions

5 reps to complete 1 set.

Precaution

It may seem a little tough for beginners. So, try doing 2 reps initially, and then gradually increase the reps and sets.

7. Shoulder Raise

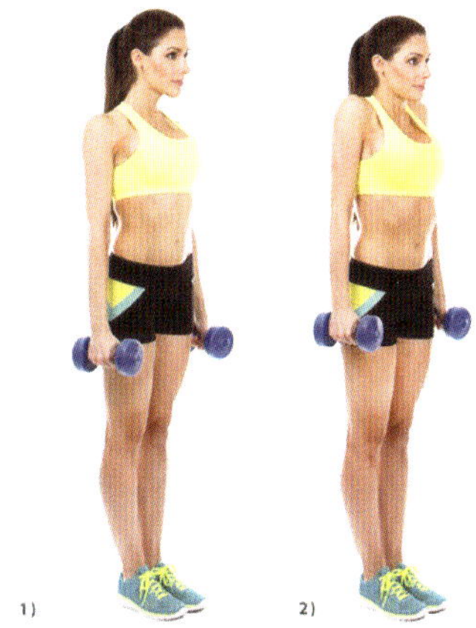

Target

Anterior deltoid, trapezius muscles, lats, and the supraspinatus.

Starting Position

Hold the dumbbells, one in each hand, and look straight ahead.

Steps To Do

1. Do not bend your elbows. Raise your shoulders and hold for 10-15 seconds.
2. Bring your hands down and relax.

Repetitions

5 reps to complete 1 set.

Precaution

Avoid doing this exercise if you have a previous shoulder injury.

8. Shoulder Extension

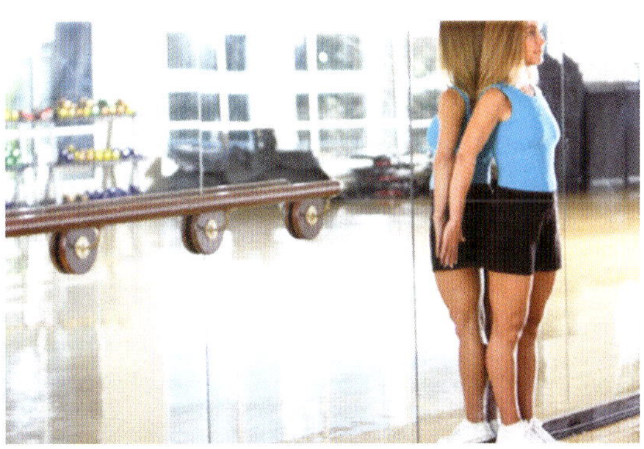

Target

Deltoids, lats, and triceps.

Starting Position

Stand straight with the support of a wall.

Steps To Do

1. Straighten your elbows while stretching your shoulders.
2. Hold for 5 seconds and release.
3. Repeat 10 times.

Repetitions

10 reps to complete 1 set.

Precaution

Keep your back straight while doing this exercise.

9. Isometric Shoulder Press

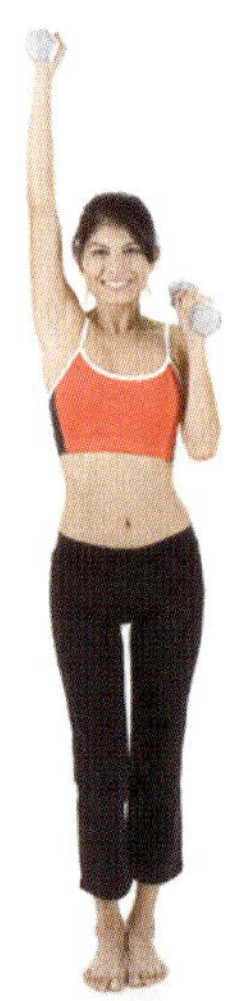

Target

Rotor cuffs, lats, triceps, and biceps.

Starting Position

Hold 2-pound dumbbells in your hands and lift them till the shoulder level. Flex your elbows so that your forearms and upper arms are at 90 degrees with each other.

Steps To Do

1. Start pressing one arm by steadily extending your arm and then bring it back to the starting position. The other arm will remain static.
2. Do the same with the other arm.

Repetitions

5 reps to complete one set on each arm.

Precaution

Maintain the 90-degree angle.

10. Isometric Shoulder Internal Rotation

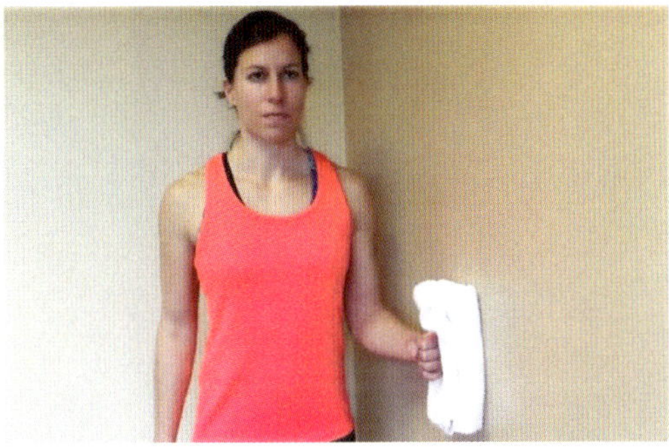

Target

Shoulders, back, forearms, and upper arms.

Starting Position

Stand upright with your elbow flexed at 90 degrees. Place a folded towel between your arm and the wall.

Steps To Do

1. Push your arm into the wall as if you are rotating your forearm outward, keeping your elbow tucked to your side.
2. Relax and repeat.

Repetitions

5 reps to complete 1 set.

Precaution

Make sure to keep your back straight during the exercise.

Isometric Exercises For The Back

11. Warrior III

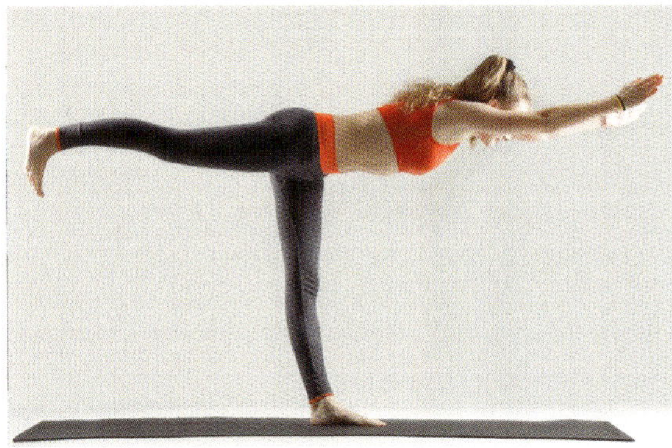

Target

Lats, shoulders, obliques, biceps, glutes, quads, and hamstrings.

Starting Position

Start in Tadasana and slowly shift your weight to your right leg.

Steps To Do

1. Start lifting the left leg slowly, bending forward at the same time.
2. Keep your back erect and spine straight the entire time.
3. Bend forward and lift your leg until your spine and the lifted leg are aligned in a straight, horizontal line.
4. Keep that balance and hold the pose for 10 seconds.
5. Slowly lower your leg. Repeat the pose with the other leg.

Repetitions

3 reps to complete 1 set.

Precaution

Take the support of a wall initially if you find it difficult to balance your body.

12. The Bridge

Target

Gluteus maximus, obliques, erector spinae, gluteus maximus, rectus abdominis, and obliques.

Starting Position

Lie down on your back on the floor. Flex your knees, keep your hands on the sides, and feet and palms flat on the ground.

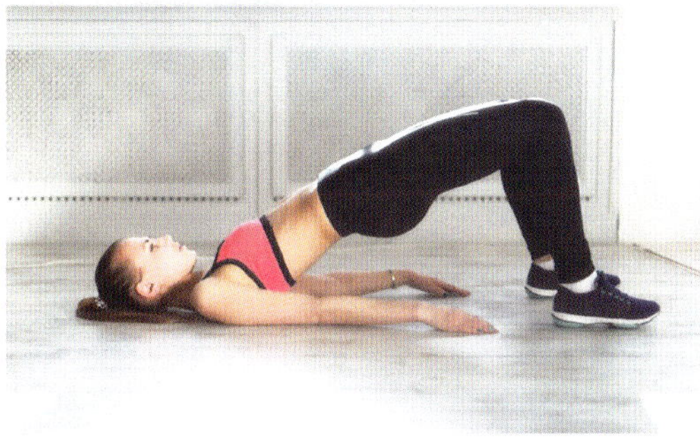

Steps To Do

1. Support your body on your feet on and palms and gently thrust your hip upwards.
2. Hold this position for 10 seconds before lowering your body back to the starting position.

Repetitions

5 reps to complete 1 set.

Precaution

Keep your head and neck straight. Look up at the ceiling while doing this exercise.

13. Back Stretch

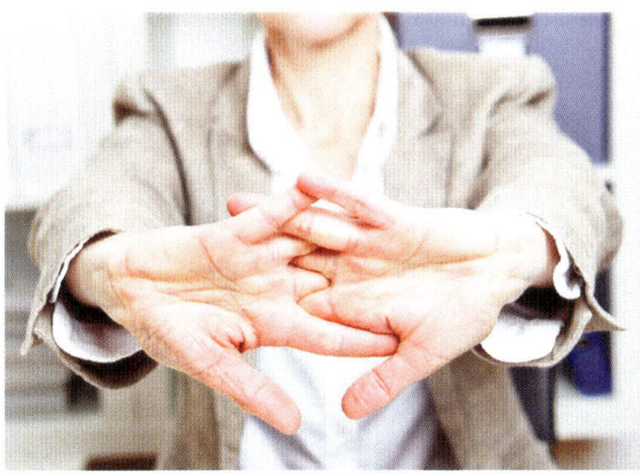

Target

Lats, obliques, chest, upper abs, shoulders, and neck.

Starting Position

Stand straight. Keep your shoulders relaxed, and hands by your side.

Steps To Do

1. Hold your arms out and interlock your hands.
2. Pull your shoulders back so that your chest pops out and your feel the stretch just below your shoulders.
3. Flex your elbows and bring your interlocked hands close to your navel.
4. Push your shoulders back and feel the middle back muscles contract. Hold it for 2 seconds and release.

Repetitions

5 reps to complete 1 set.

Precaution

Exhale as you pull your shoulders back.

14. Towel Row

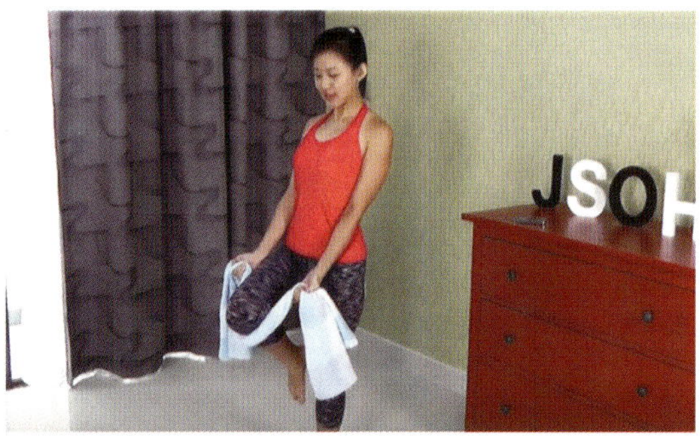

Target

Rhomboids, glutes, lats, shoulders, and biceps.

Starting Position

Stand straight with your legs shoulder-width apart. Hold the ends of a towel in your hands. Flex one knee and put it over the towel.

Steps To Do

1. Raise your arms towards your shoulders as much as possible so that you can feel the stretch in your back, arms, and glutes.
2. Hold it for 30 seconds before releasing and reverting to the starting position.

Repetitions

5 reps to complete 1 set.

Precaution

Sit straight while doing this exercise.

Isometric Exercises For The Legs

15. Wall Sit

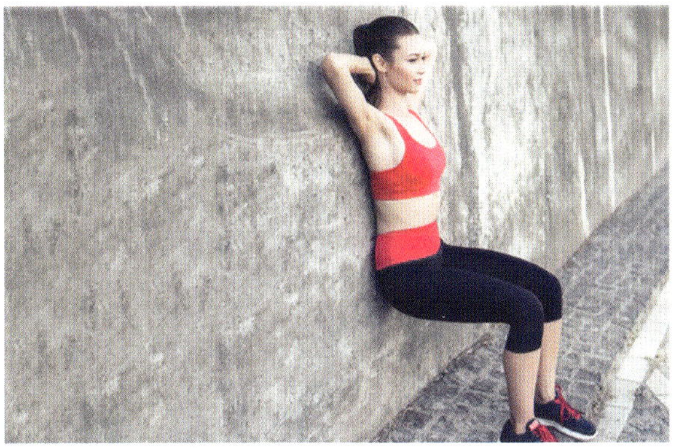

Target

Hamstrings, quads, calves, and lower back.

Starting Position

Stand with your back against a wall.

Steps To Do

1. Flex your knees and lower your body as you would while squatting.
2. Hold the position for 5-7 seconds and release.
3. Repeat this 10 times. Increase the hold time gradually.

Repetitions

5 reps to complete 1 set.

Precaution

Make sure you keep your back against the wall at all times.

16. Isometric Quads

Target

Quadriceps or the front of your thighs.

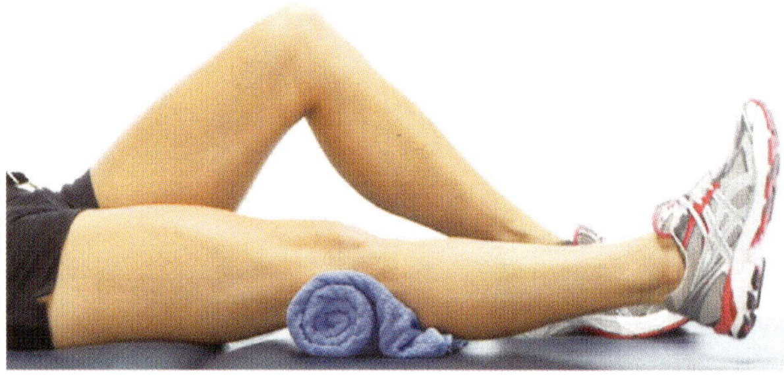

Starting Position

Lie down flat on your back. Keep one leg straight and one knee flexed, and the foot flat on the ground. Keep a rolled towel or a cushion underneath your straight leg's knee.

Steps To Do

1. Once you rest your knee, raise it to form a bend and hold for 5 seconds.
2. Rest it back on the cushion and repeat the procedure with the other knee.
3. Do this for each knee with at least 15 repetitions each.

Repetitions

15 reps to complete 1 set.

Precaution

Lie down on a flat and sturdy surface.

17. Ankle Press

Target

Peroneal muscles and calves.

Starting Position

Lie down on your back and hold a pillow between your ankles.

Steps To Do

1. Press the pillow as hard as you can till you touch the other ankle.
2. Hold it for 10 seconds.

Repetitions

15 reps to complete 1 set.

Precaution

Do not use a hard object as you may hurt your ankle.

18. Weighted Calf Raises

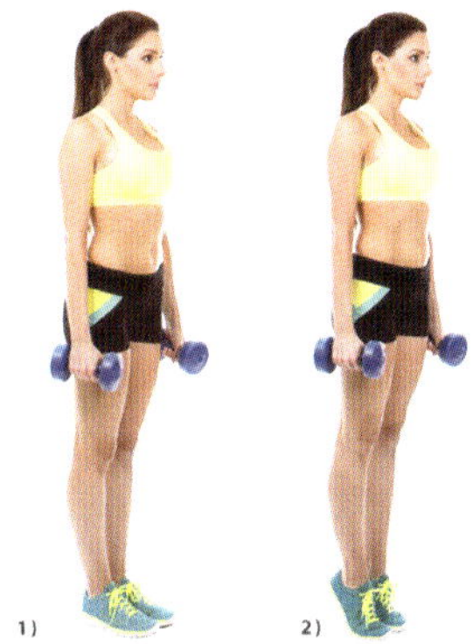

Target

Calves, glutes, and arms.

Starting Position

Stand straight and hold a dumbbell in each hand by your side with the arms straight.

Steps To Do

1. Raise your heels off the floor and balance yourself on the balls of your feet.
2. Hold for 10 seconds.
3. Another version is to continue doing calf raises while holding the weight in your hands.

Repetitions

10 reps to complete 1 set.

Precaution

Use weights that are not too light or too heavy.

19. Isometric Knee Exercise

Target

Knees, quads, hamstrings, adductors, and calves.

Starting Position

Sit on the floor with your legs extended in front of you.

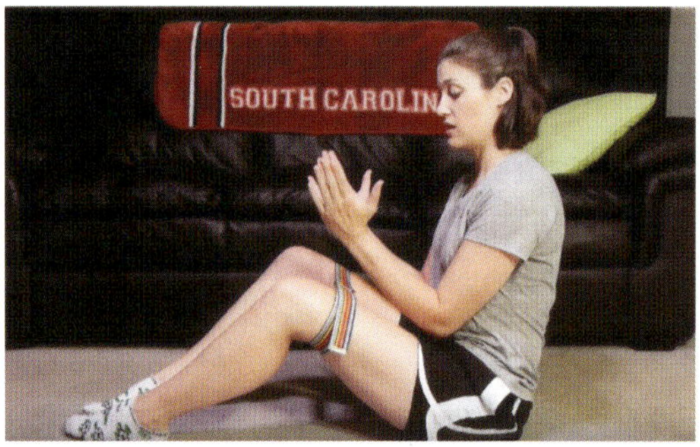

Steps To Do

1. Keep one leg straight and flex the other knee. Keep the foot flat on the floor.
2. Place a rolled towel underneath your straight leg's knee.
3. Push your knee down as hard as you can. This will work on your quads.
4. Hold it for 3 seconds, relax, and repeat 10 times.
5. Flex your straight leg and push your heel down to the ground.
6. Hold it for 3 seconds, relax, and repeat 10 times.
7. Now, keep both your feet flat on the ground and the knees flexed.
8. Use a belt (not a resistance band) and tie it around your thighs.
9. Push both your legs out. Hold for 3 seconds, relax, and repeat 10 times.
10. Grab a medicine ball and hold it between your knees.
11. Squeeze in your legs so that you feel the burn in your inner thighs.
12. Hold it for 3 seconds, relax, and repeat.

Repetitions

5 reps to complete 1 set.

Precaution

If you do not have a medicine ball or a towel, use a pillow to do the exercises.

20. Static Lunge

Target

Quads, hamstrings. lower back, and glutes.

Starting Position

Stand with all the muscles in your body tensed, your core tight, and shoulders back.

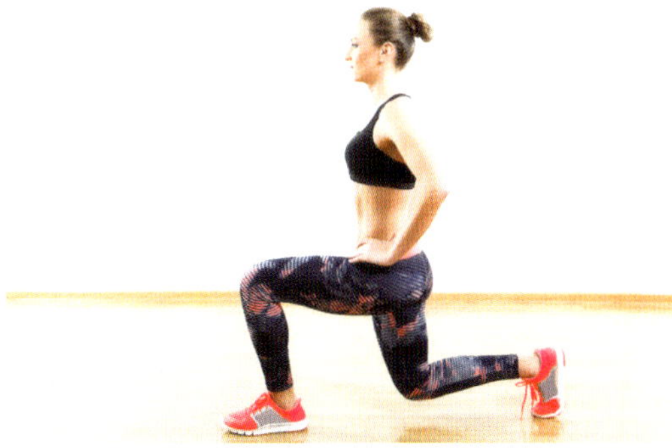

Steps To Do

1. Split and take your left leg back in a lunge.
2. Lower yourself into as deep a lunge as you can without touching your bent knee to the ground. Ideally, lower yourself until you are just inches above the ground.
3. Hold this pose for 10 seconds and repeat with the other leg.
4. To intensify the exercise, grab a heavy dumbbell in each hand.

Repetitions

10 reps to complete 1 set.

Precaution

Do not try to overtrain. You must build the strength gradually to avoid injuries.

21. Squat Hold

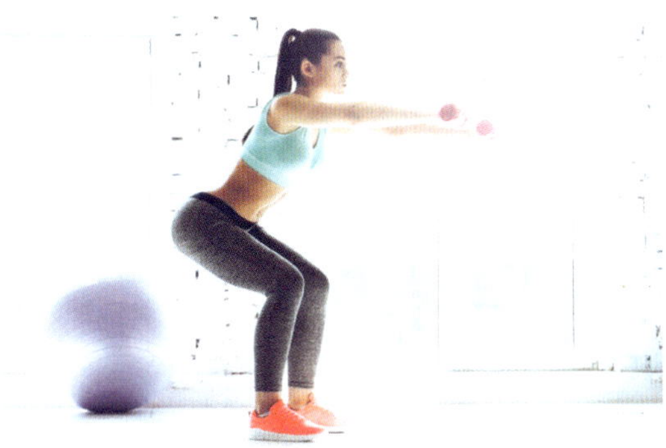

Target

Adductors, glutes, quads, hamstrings, and lower back.

Starting Position

Stand straight with your legs shoulder-width apart.

Steps To Do

1. For a mid-squat hold, lower yourself into a squat and stop when you reach about the middle of your length as if you are sitting on a chair. Hold yourself in the pose for 10 seconds.
2. For a deep squat, lower yourself into a complete squat to the ground with your knees up to your chest and your butt inches off the floor. Hold the pose for 15 seconds.

Repetitions

10 reps to complete 1 set.

Precaution

When you squat, make sure your back is straight and your knees do not overshoot your feet.

Isometric Exercises For The Arms

22. Wall Push-up

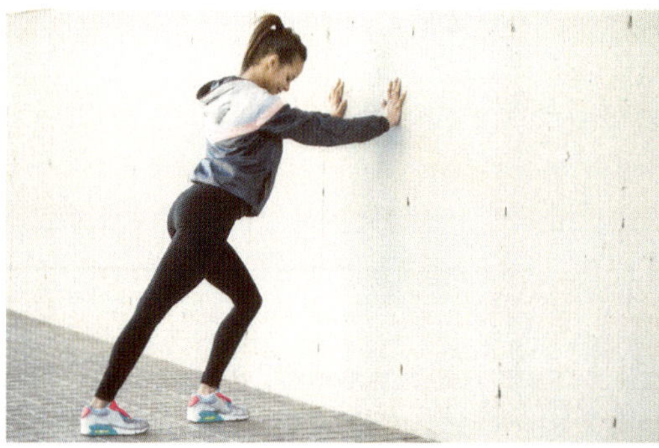

Target

Biceps, triceps, shoulders, lats, and chest.

Starting Position

Place your hands on the wall, shoulder-width apart.

Steps To Do

1. Lean on the wall, supporting your body on your toes, and keep your palms on the wall.
2. Push as hard as you can.
3. Keep pushing with the same force for 15 seconds. Relax.

Repetitions

5 reps to complete 1 set.

Precaution

Keep your back straight while doing this exercise.

23. Isometric Towel Curls

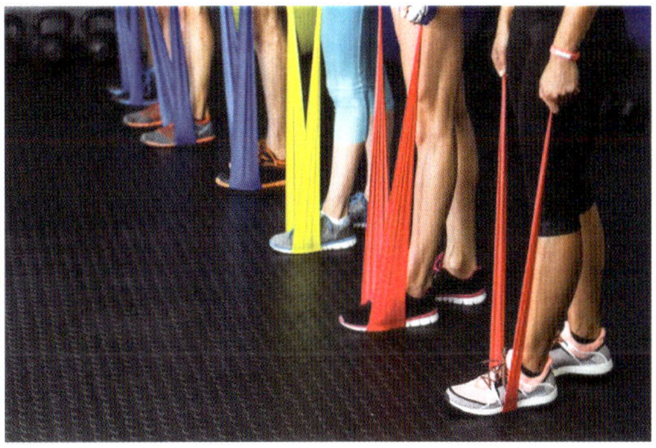

Target

Biceps

Starting Position

Take a long towel and hold both its ends in your hands. Hold the lower portion of the towel with one of your feet.

Steps To Do

1. Try pulling up the towel. You will feel the stretch in your arms.
2. Hold it for 3 seconds, relax, and repeat 10 times.

Repetitions

10 reps to complete 1 set.

Precaution

Keep your back straight and flex your knees slightly while doing this exercise.

24. Body Weight Resisted Tricep Push Extensions

Target

Triceps

Starting Position

Stand straight with your feet hip-width apart. Raise your hands above your head and clasp them together.

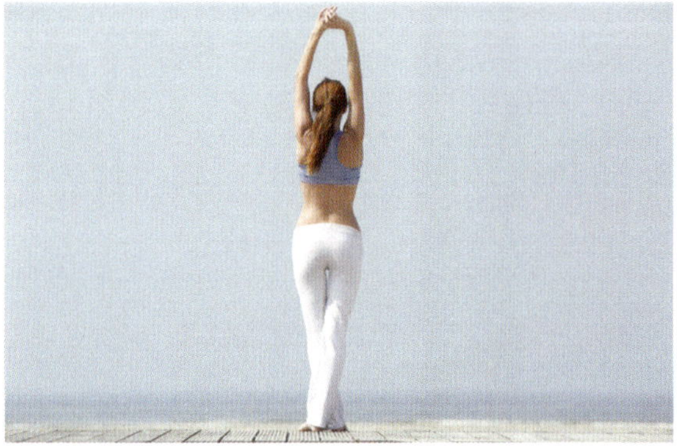

Steps To Do

1. Raise your right arm and bend your left arm slightly to resist the right arm.
2. Squeeze hard to feel the stretch in your triceps.
3. Hold it for 10 seconds, relax, and repeat 10 times.
4. Do it with the other hand.

Repetitions

5 reps to complete one set.

Precaution

Keep your shoulders relaxed and core engaged while doing this exercise.

25. Barbell Isometric Curls

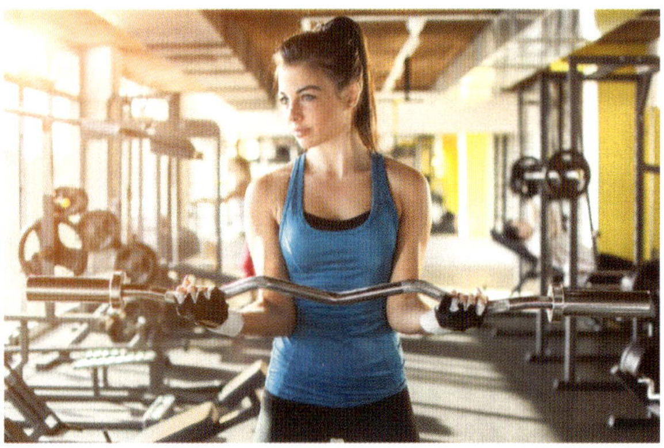

Target

Forearms, biceps, triceps, and shoulders.

Starting Position

Hold a barbell. Stand straight with your feet shoulder-width apart and core engaged.

Steps To Do

1. Lift the barbell till your hands reach your shoulders.
2. Hold this position for 20 seconds and feel the contraction.
3. Relax and lower the barbell to the starting position.

Repetitions

5 reps to complete 1 set.

Precaution

Make sure to use weights that are neither too heavy nor too light.

Isometric Exercises For The Neck

26. Neck Stretch

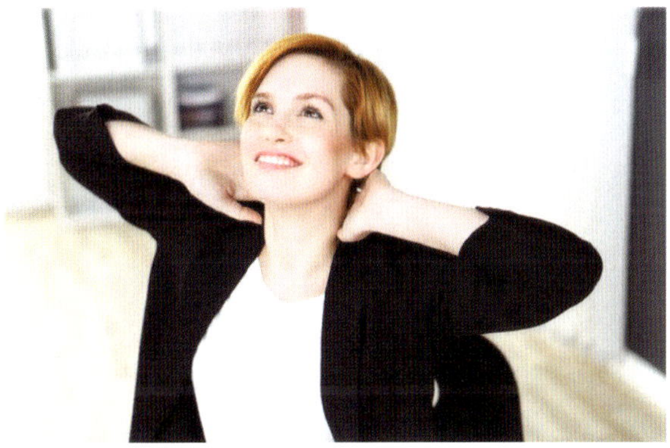

Target

Neck muscles

Starting Position

Place both your palms on your forehead and stand straight with your feet hip-width apart.

Steps To Do

1. Push your forehead towards your palms and use them to resist that force. Hold it for 5-8 seconds for 3 repetitions.
2. Put your hands behind your head. Push your head towards your hands and vice versa. Hold it for 5-8 seconds for 3 repetitions.
3. Put your right hand on the right side of your head. Push your head towards your hand and vice versa. Hold it for 5-8 seconds for 3 repetitions. Do it for the left side as well.

4. Put your right palm on the sides of your cheeks. Push your hands inwards and use your face to resist that force. Hold it for 5-8 seconds for 3 repetitions. Do it for the left side as well.

Repetitions

3 reps to complete 1 set.

Precaution

Avoid hurting yourself by pressing your head too hard.

Isometric Exercise For The Glutes

27. Hip Adduction

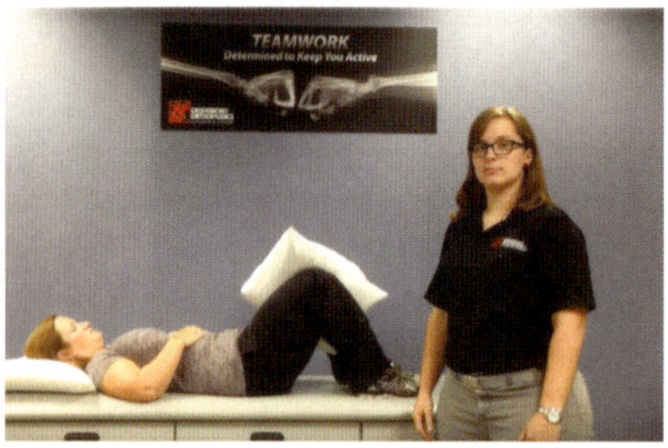

Target

Glutes, adductors, and lower back.

Starting Position

Lie down on your back, flex your knees, and keep your feet flat on the ground.

Steps To Do

1. Hold a pillow with your thighs.
2. Press it as hard as possible, ensuring the pressure from both the sides is at the same time.
3. Release your thighs without letting the pillow fall. During the course of pressing and releasing, your breathing must be evenly controlled.

Repetitions

5 reps to complete 1 set.

Precaution

Lie down on a completely flat and sturdy surface.

Isometric Exercise For The Chest

28. Chest Squeeze

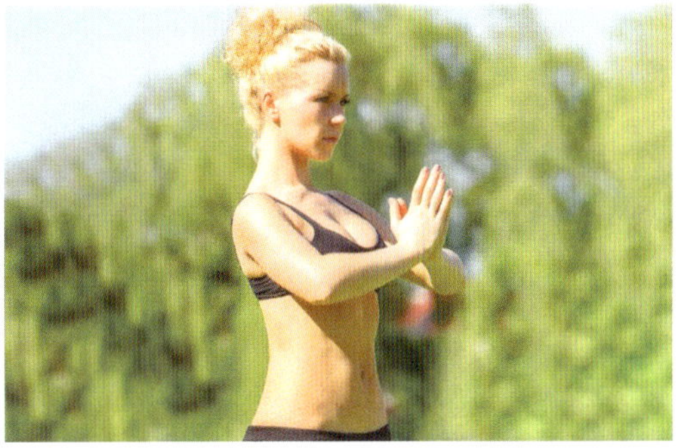

Target

Pectoralis major and pectoralis minor muscles.

Starting Position

Stand straight with your legs hip-width apart.

Steps To Do

1. Put your palms together and press them. Hold for 10 seconds.
2. Lift your right leg and balance. Hold for 10 seconds.
3. Lower your right leg and lift your left leg. Hold for 10 seconds.

Repetitions

5 reps to complete 1 set.

Precaution

Keep your back straight while doing this exercise.

Benefits of Isometric Exercises

Practicing isometric exercises offers various benefits to your body. They are:

- Isometric exercises help in strengthening and conditioning the muscles.
- They strengthen the dormant muscle tissues on isolated muscles.
- They improve one's control over the body.
- Improve body posture and spine alignment.
- Help prevent injury.

- These exercises are used in injury rehabilitation.
- Help in the development of lean muscles.
- Improve bone density and make them strong.
- Increase resistance power and endurance ability.
- These exercises activate all the major units in the body.
- They can be done anywhere and anytime.
- Most isometric exercises do not require any equipment, or at the most, a set of dumbbells is enough.
- Help in graceful aging, keeping the body posture straight and erect even in old age.
- These exercises can also be done by the elderly and are considered good for them.

Lower Body Weight Training

Squat

Squats are a compound movement – which means it's a movement that uses more than one joint (your hip and knee joints) to complete.

A simple bodyweight squat workout uses almost every muscle group in the body – and if you add a dumbbell or barbell into the equation, they use *every single* major muscle group to complete.

Squats will help strengthen your entire body, both your bones and your muscles (and your knees!), and increase flexibility.

Because of the utilization of a large amount of muscle groups, they cause your body to increase our anabolic hormone production (in turn, helping us lose fat and gain muscle).

Increasing the strength in your knees and hips (and entire body) reduces your chance of injury while doing both athletic movements and everyday life things (such as shoveling the driveway or standing up and sitting down).

The Bodyweight Squat

Become a bodyweight squat pro, and you'll be ready to move on to weighted squats in no time! Just follow these steps.

1. Stand with feet a little wider than shoulder-width apart, hips stacked over knees, and knees over ankles.

2. Roll the shoulders back and down away from the ears. Note: Allowing the back to round (like a turtle's shell) will cause unnecessary stress on the lower back. It's important to maintain a neutral spine throughout the movement.

3. Extend arms out straight so they are parallel with the ground, palms facing down (like your hands are on someone's shoulders at a 7th grade dance). Or, if it's more comfortable, pull elbows close to the body, palms facing each other and thumbs pointing up.

4. Initiate the movement by inhaling and unlocking the hips, slightly bringing them back. Keep sending hips backward as the knees begin to bend.

5. While the butt starts to stick out, make sure the chest and shoulders stay upright, and the back stays straight. Keep the head facing forward with eyes straight ahead for a neutral spine.

6. The best squats are the deepest ones your mobility allows. Optimal squat depth would be your hips sinking below the knees. Squatting onto a box until the butt gently taps it will be a reminder to squat low.

7. Engage core and, with bodyweight in the heels, explode back up to standing, driving through heels. Imagine the feet are spreading the floor without actually moving the feet.

Goblet Squat

This squat (sadly) does not include a goblet full of wine (though we've found no studies disproving the effectiveness). Instead, hold a kettlebell, dumbbell, or medicine ball at the sternum (center of the chest). With a slight bend in the knees, drop into a squat, going straight down and then standing straight up (do not reach back with the butt as you would for a bodyweight squat). When performing a goblet squat, drop the elbows between the legs inside the knees for a full range of motion. Goblet squats are great for beginners (and also experienced lifters) since they keep us from leaning forward (holding weight in front of the chest makes for a stable position).

Back Squat

Squats are much more challenging with a barbell, so if it's your first time, it's best to ask for a trainer's guidance. For back squats, the weight rests on the traps (in one of two positions: low or high), where it's generally easier to squat a heavier load. Hands should be facing forward, along the same plane as the shoulders, with elbows pointing down to the ground (arms will form a "W" along the bar). Keep hips back, and follow the same form for a bodyweight squat. The back squat is different from the bodyweight squat in one important way: breathing. When you're squatting a barbell, inhale before you descend, hold your breath for the squat, and exhale only once you've returned to standing.

Front Squat

The front squat requires getting comfortable with the front rack position. When front-squatting with a barbell, this means resting the barbell just above the clavicles, right on the neck (the ends of the bar will rest on the shoulders if they're wide enough) and laying on the fingertips, with elbows up and pointed out and triceps parallel to the ground. While it may seem unstable to hold the bar with just the fingertips, the collarbone is a solid shelf for the bar, so the hands are only needed to prevent the bar from rolling. As long as the elbows stay up, extending straight out from the shoulders, the bar will be secure. For the descent in a front squat, the body will stay signifcantly more upright than it would in a bodyweight or back squat.

Do not reach back with the butt (as you would with a back or bodyweight squat), as this will angle the body forward, making it difficult to stand the weight up. A great way to maintain an upright position is to think about keeping the elbows up and pointing forward throughout the movement.

The front squat can also be done with dumbbells. With one in each hand (palms facing in), rest a dumbbell lightly on each shoulder. Execute the squat, keeping the triceps raised and elbows up and pointed out.

Leg Press

The leg press is a unique movement. For an exercise with quite a short range of motion, it stimulates the quads, glutes and hamstrings to their maximum potential.

Place your feet on the pad shoulder-width apart. Ensure there is a slight outward angle to your toe position so they aren't pointing straight forwards. If you want to place more stress on the glutes, position your feet high on the pad. If greater quad growth is more of a goal, position your feet towards the bottom.

Straighten your legs and release the leg press handles. Keep your entire back, particularly the lower portion, firmly set against the seat. This reduces any strain placed on the lower back and keeps it on the glutes.

Keeping your feet set, lower your legs towards your chest – being careful not to bounce your knees off your chest – then press up again. Don't fully lock your legs out at the knee – this maintains muscular tension on the quads and doesn't risk a knee injury.

Leg Press Pros

Because resistance machines such as the leg press only allow movement in a fixed pattern, they're great for beginners or people coming back from an injury, who need to master a correct and safe movement pattern before advancing to the more challenging barbell and dumbbell leg lifts.

They are also useful for people who want to isolate a specific muscle, in this case the quads, hamstrings and glutes. That's because the fixed movement of the machine doesn't require the stabilising muscles – nearly always the weak link that limits the amount of weight that can be moved – so you can lift heavy in the safest possible way to maximise muscle growth. You can also adjust the weight you are lifting very quickly.

Leg Press Cons

Resistance machines don't require the activation or engagement of any of the important stabilising muscles, which means using them at the expense of free weights can lead to muscular imbalances and an injury-prone body. With the leg press, while your major lower-body muscles will get thoroughly taxed, those crucial smaller supporting muscles of the hips, knees and ankles aren't fully engaged, so they won't be worked as hard as is necessary to develop all-round lower-body strength and joint and muscle stability.

Upper Body Weight Training

Pectorals

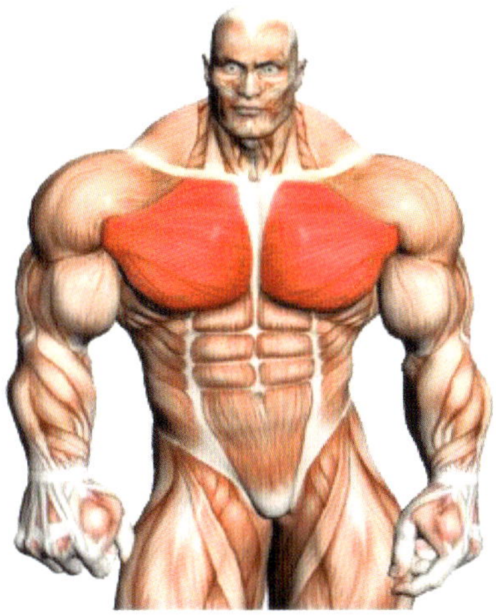

The pectoralis major covers the upper chest connecting the sternum, the cartilage of the first 6 ribs and the white sheath of the obliques and the rectus abdominis to the humerus bone of the upper arm.

The pectoralis major (from Latin: pectus, breast) is a thick, fan-shaped muscle, situated at the chest (anterior) of the human body.

It makes up the bulk of the chest muscles in the male and lies under the breast in the female. Underneath the pectoralis major is the pectoralis minor, a thin, triangular muscle. In sports as well as bodybuilding, the pectoral muscles may colloquially be referred to as "pecs".

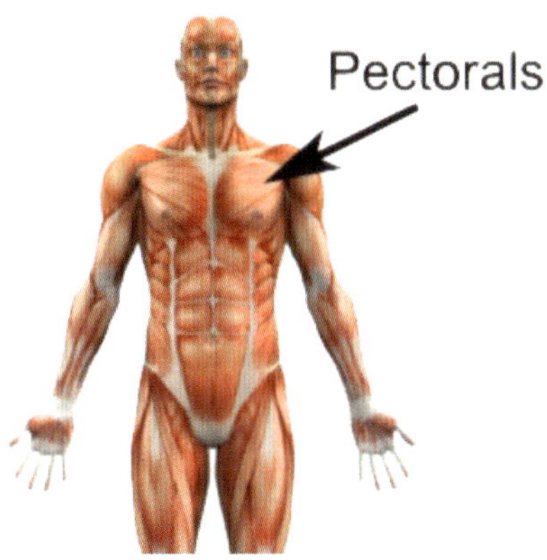

The pectoralis major muscle is a large muscle in the upper chest, fanning across the chest from the shoulder to the breastbone. The two pectoralis major muscles, commonly referred to as the "pecs," are the muscles that create the bulk of the chest. A developed pectoralis major is most evident in males, as the breasts of a female typically hide the pectoral muscles. A second pectoral muscle, the pectoralis minor, lies beneath the pectoralis major. The pectorals are predominantly used to control the movement of the arm, with the contractions of the pectoralis major pulling on the humerus to create lateral, vertical, or rotational motion. The pectorals also play a part in deep inhalation, pulling the ribcage to create room for the lungs to expand.

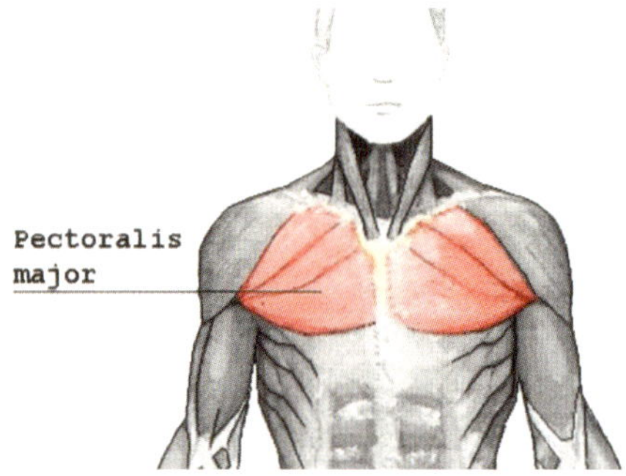

Pectoralis Muscles of Chest Exercises

Dumbbells Bench Press

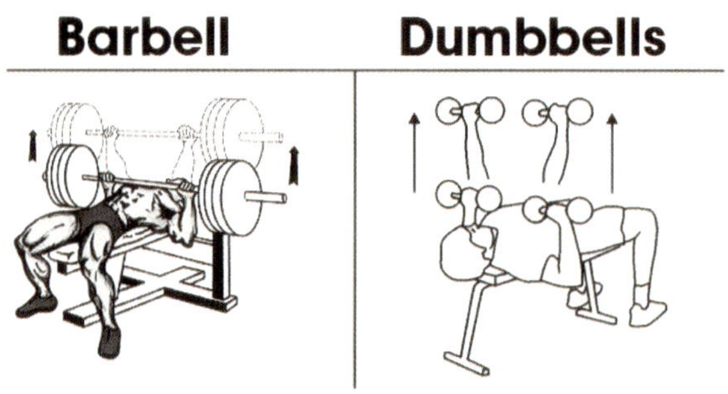

Proper Bench Press form starts lying on a Bench with your feet on the floor. Unrack the bar with straight arms. Lower it to your mid-chest. Press it back up until you've locked your elbows. Keep your butt on the bench. Bench Press sets of five reps every Strong Lifts 5×5 workout A. The Bench Press is a full body, compound exercise. It works your chest, shoulders and triceps most. It's the most effective exercise to gain upper-body strength and muscle because it's the upper-body exercise you'll lift most weight on (more than Overhead Press). The bigger your bench, the bigger your chest. To avoid shoulder pain, tuck your elbows 75° when you lower the bar. Don't try to stretch your chest by flaring your elbows 90° out. You'll impinge your shoulders if your upper-arms are perpendicular to your torso at the bottom. Tuck your elbows 75° to Bench Press pain-free. Unlike the Squat or Deadlift, the bar doesn't move in a vertical line when you Bench Press with proper form. It moves diagonally from your mid-chest over your shoulders. This is the safest way to Bench Press for your shoulders. It's also the most effective way to Bench Press heavy.

Pec Deck Fly

Single-joint exercises like the pec-deck flye are typically done after heavy multijoint moves (at various angles) in your chest workout. The pec deck allows you to destroy your outer and inner chest fibers with pinpoint accuracy. For variety, you can also do this move at the beginning of your routine to pre-exhaust the chest. Most always done last, it's a great way to flush and pump the fibers of the pectoral muscles.

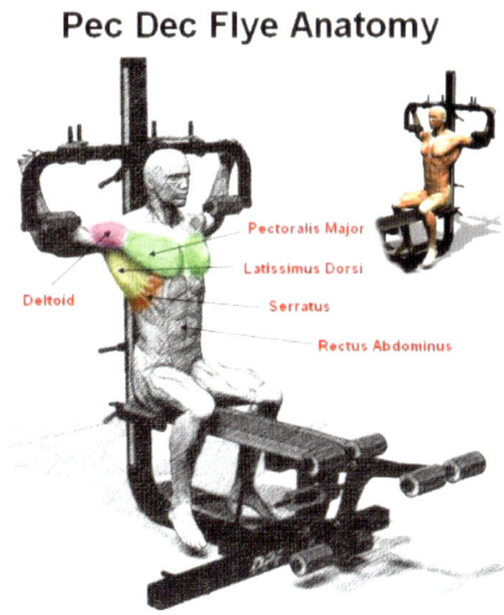

Chest Press Machine

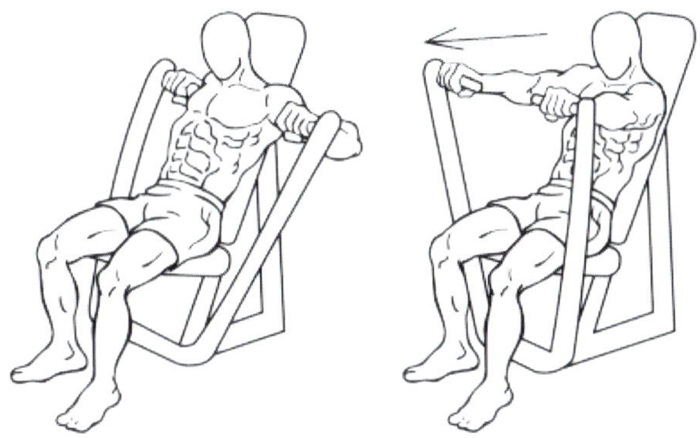

- Sit down on the Chest Press Machine and select the weight.
- Step on the lever provided by the machine since it will help you to bring the handles forward so that you can grab the handles and fully extend the arms.
- Grab the handles with a palms-down grip and lift your elbows so that your upper arms are parallel to the floor to the sides of your torso. Tip: Your forearms will be pointing forward since you are grabbing the handles. Once you bring the handles forward and extend the arms you will be at the starting position.
- Now bring the handles back towards you as you breathe in.
- Push the handles away from you as you flex your pecs and you breathe out. Hold the contraction for a second before going back to the starting position.
- Repeat for the recommended amount of reps.
- When finished step on the lever again and slowly get the handles back to their original place.

Variations

You can use free weights (barbells and dumbbells) to perform this exercise on a regular bench. Alternatively, you can use the pulley machine as well.

Incline Dumbbell Flyes

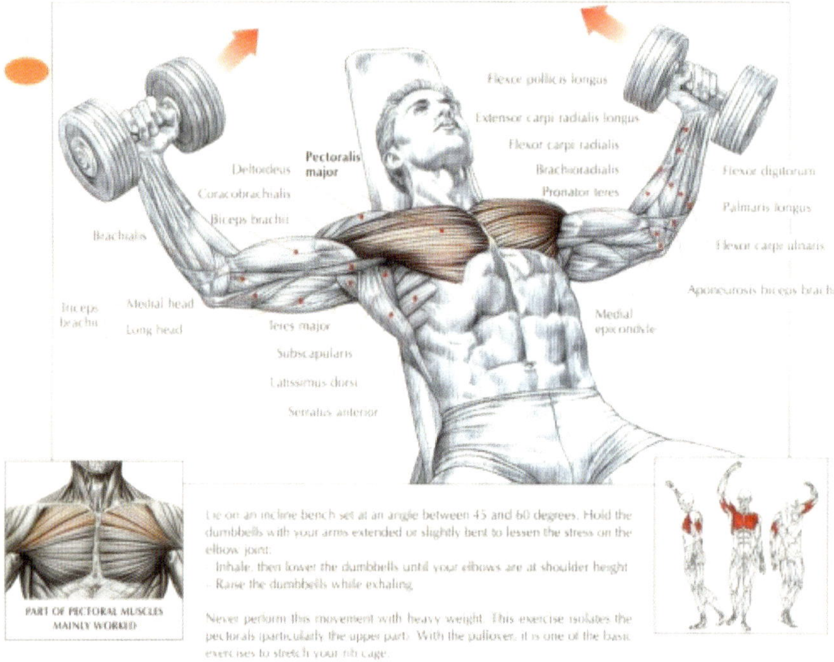

- Hold a dumbbell on each hand and lie on an incline bench that is set to an incline angle of no more than 30 degrees.
- Extend your arms above you with a slight bend at the elbows.
- Now rotate the wrists so that the palms of your hands are facing you. Tip: The pinky fingers should be next to each other. This will be your starting position.
- As you breathe in, start to slowly lower the arms to the side while keeping the arms extended and while rotating the wrists until the palms of the hand are facing each other. Tip: At the end of the movement the arms will be by your side with the palms facing the ceiling.
- As you exhale start to bring the dumbbells back up to the starting position by reversing the motion and rotating the hands so that the pinky fingers are next to each other again. Tip: Keep in mind that the movement will only happen at the shoulder joint and at the wrist. There is no motion that happens at the elbow joint.
- Repeat for the recommended amount of repetitions.

Variations

You can perform regular flyes and also twisting flyes where your initial position starts with the thumbs facing each other instead of the pinky.

Parallel bars are an awesome bodyweight training tool for practicing your hand balancing, and this week we've got two incredible exercises for you to try out: the L-Sit to High Hip Tuck; and the L-Sit to Straddle Press-Up Handstand. Whether you are a gymnast, bar athlete or general bodyweight enthusiast, Parallels are an excellent place to work on your strength, coordination, and stabilization while building some seriously cool skills!

Incline Barbell Bench Press

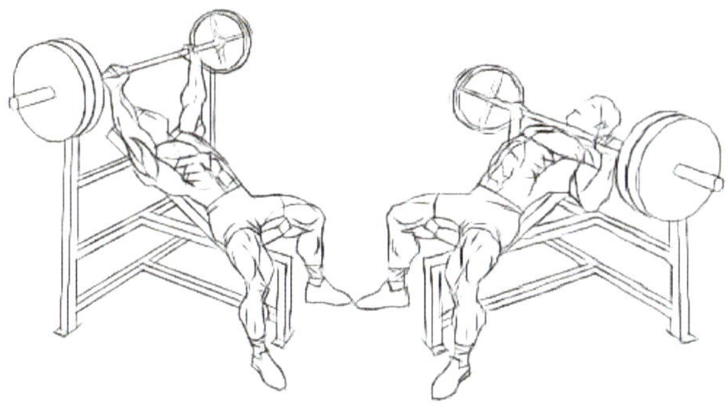

The incline barbell bench press is a great way to add variety to your pressing routine and to hit muscle groups from different angles leading to new growth. Taking nothing away from the barbell bench press, the incline press can allow you to really focus on your upper and inner chest muscles and shoulders. The strictness of the exercise takes away any arching of the back to shorten your range of motion and decreases the help from leg drive. Let's take a look at how this exercise can help you round out your physique and bust through any plateaus you might have with the flat bench press.

Decline Barbell Bench Press

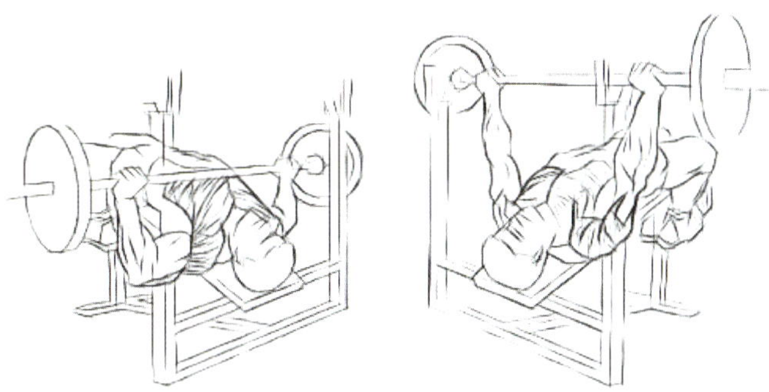

1. Secure your legs at the end of the decline bench and slowly lay down on the bench.
2. Using a medium width grip (a grip that creates a 90-degree angle in the middle of the movement between the forearms and the upper arms), lift the bar from the rack and hold it straight over you with your arms locked. The arms should be perpendicular to the floor. This will be your starting position. Tip: In order to protect your rotator cuff, it is best if you have a spotter help you lift the barbell off the rack.
3. As you breathe in, come down slowly until you feel the bar on your lower chest.

4. After a second pause, bring the bar back to the starting position as you breathe out and push the bar using your chest muscles. Lock your arms and squeeze your chest in the contracted position, hold for a second and then start coming down slowly again. Tip: It should take at least twice as long to go down than to come up).

5. Repeat the movement for the prescribed amount of repetitions.

6. When you are done, place the bar back in the rack.

Flat Barbell Bench Press

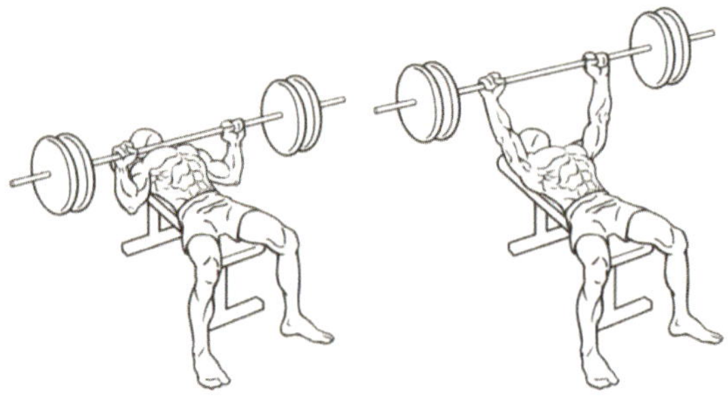

1. Lie back on a flat bench. Using a medium width grip (a grip that creates a 90-degree angle in the middle of the movement between the forearms and the upper arms), lift the bar from the rack and hold it straight over you with your arms locked. This will be your starting position.

2. From the starting position, breathe in and begin coming down slowly until the bar touches your middle chest.

3. After a brief pause, push the bar back to the starting position as you breathe out. Focus on pushing the bar using your chest muscles. Lock your arms and squeeze your chest in the contracted position at the top of the motion, hold for a second and then start coming down slowly again. Tip: Ideally, lowering the weight should take about twice as long as raising it.

4. Repeat the movement for the prescribed amount of repetitions.

5. When you are done, place the bar back in the rack.

Parallel Bar Dips

When it comes to building lower pectorals, triceps and frontal deltoids, dips are without doubt one the best exercises one can use. They are seldom used nowadays and the reasons are plain to see: one should be able to handle their own bodyweight for reps – unless one have access to one of those fancy-dan machines that allow them to dip (or chin) with less than body weight.

A correctly done dip has two distinct rep-stroke lengths, two levels: drop down until upper arms are parallel to the floor or go all the way down as far as you can. Either depth works the triceps exquisitely, assuming you lockout hard at the top of every rep and hold that flexion for a beat before lower yet again. The parallel tricep dip is a tricep isolation movement with some slight pectoral and front deltoid stimulation.

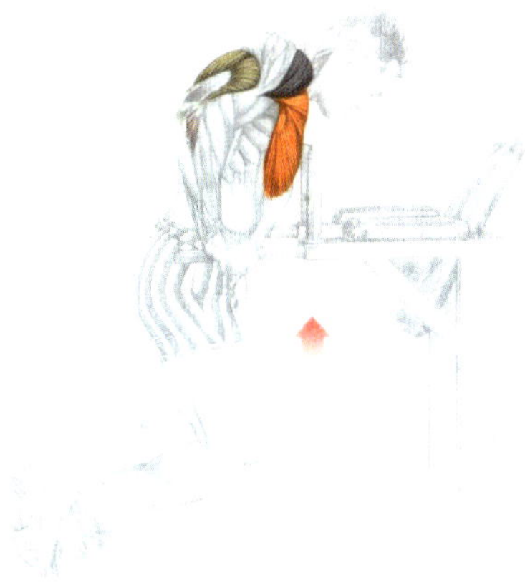

Triceps

The muscles on the back of the arms are called the triceps. In anatomy, the technical term is actually "triceps brachii", which is Latin for three-headed muscle. Though this seems to make your triceps sound like some kind of fairy-tale monster, the reason for this name is that the triceps are comprised of three different muscle bundles on the outside, middle, and inside of the back of your arms.

Because the triceps has three different muscles, simply doing one exercise is typically not enough to tone the back of your arms. Instead, you need to come at that three-headed monster from as many angles as possible, using a variety of exercises and hand positions.

Exercises for the Triceps

The triceps are too often neglected, even though they are an obvious opposing muscle to the biceps, and even though we exercise the biceps more often.

Two of the most common triceps exercises are:

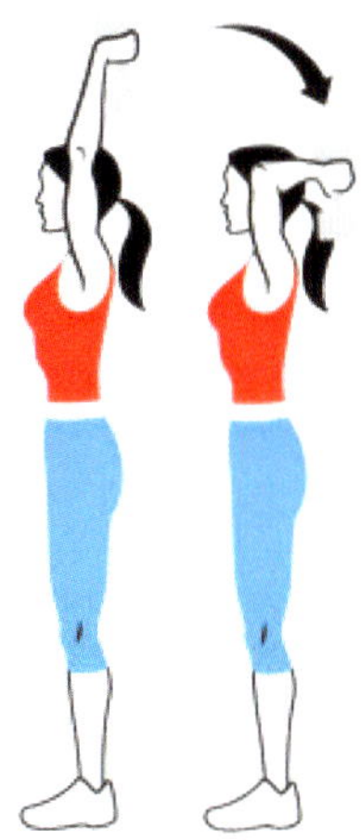

- Tricep or Overhead Extension: Hold on to the end of the dumbbell with both hands. Begin with your arms straight and your feet hip-width apart. Keep your upper arms still while bending your elbows to lower the weight slowly behind your head. Then straighten your arms and return to the starting position. Attempt 8-12 repetitions, but do not over-exert. Begin with fewer repetitions and, as time passes and the muscle gets stronger, you'll be able to have more repetitions.

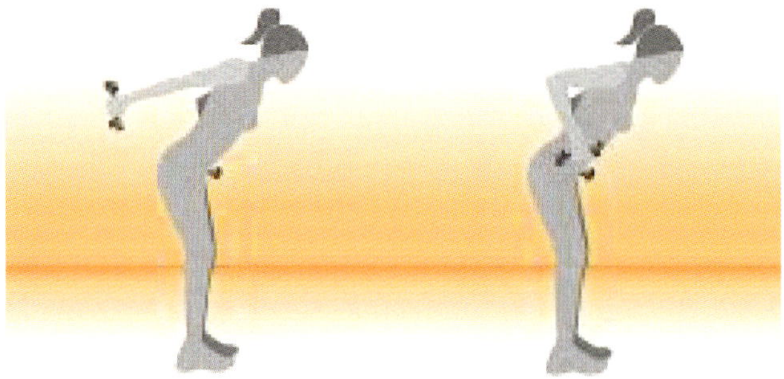

- Tricep Kickback: Place one foot forward or stand with feet hip-width apart. Hold the weights in your hands, palm facing inward. Bend the elbows and place the weights at waist-level. Bend forward slightly at the hips and then straighten the arm to the back and return to the waist (you can do both arms at the same time, or one arm at a time). Repeat as many times as you are able, usually 8-12 repetitions.

Biceps (Front of Arms)

The *biceps brachii* (usually referred to as "the bicep") was given that name because it has two heads. Most people know that it lies on the upper arm between the shoulder and the elbow. Both heads originate on the scapula and together they attach to the upper forearm. Even though the biceps cross both the shoulder and elbow, its primary function is at the elbow where it flexes and/or turns the forearm.

The biceps is attached to the arm bones by tough connective tissues called tendons. The tendons that connect the biceps muscle to the shoulder joint in two places are called the proximal biceps tendons. The tendon that attaches the biceps muscle to the forearm bones (radius and ulna) is called the distal biceps tendon. When the biceps contracts, it pulls the forearm up and rotates it outward.

The biceps can be strengthened using weight and resistance training. It is a very visible muscle — people (and cartoon characters) will bend their elbow and "show off" their biceps, especially if there is considerable bulk developed.

Older adults, however, are not exercising their biceps to gain bulk or to compete in the next Olympics. The biceps are particularly important to older adults if they fall, as their arms usually are used for support, and the stronger those muscles are, the better. Strong biceps will also help you to do daily chores: carrying groceries, scrubbing a pot, cleaning the shower.

Biceps Conditions

Biceps strain: A pulled biceps results from overstretching and tearing some of the biceps muscle fibers and/or tendons. Pain and sometimes swelling are the usual symptoms.

Proximal biceps tendon rupture: This is when one of the two biceps tendons in the shoulder is torn away from the bone. Sudden shoulder pain and an odd-shaped bulge in the biceps are symptoms.

Distal biceps tendon rupture: A tear of the biceps tendon at the forearm is unusual. Sudden pain over the front of the elbow and forearm weakness are symptoms.

Proximal biceps tendinitis (tendonitis): Repeated use of the biceps or problems in the shoulder can irritate the proximal biceps tendon. Pain in the shoulder and biceps is the main symptom.

Biceps contracture: The biceps becomes permanently contracted, with the elbow bent. Biceps contracture may occur after a severe stroke.

Exercises for the Biceps

Three common exercises for the biceps, using free weights (how heavy is your choice, but older adults often use 1, 2, or 5 pounds), are:

Hammer Curl: Place weights in hand with arms fully extended and palms turned in. Lift weights by bending the elbow and bringing the lower arm forward. Go all the way to the "top" (almost touching the upper arm). Return to the starting position. Do movements slowly, and breathe throughout.

Bicep Curl: Place weights in hand with arms fully extended and palms turned forward. Lift weights by bending the elbow and bringing the lower arm forward. Go all the way to the "top" (almost touching the upper arm). Return to the starting position. Do movements slowly, and breathe throughout.

Zottman Curl: Begin with weights in the same position as for a Bicep Curl. Lift weights by bending the elbow and bringing the lower arm forward and up. Go close to the upper arm, but do not touch. At the "top", turn the weights so that your palm faces down. Then slowly lower the arm to the starting position. Before beginning the next repetition, turn the palms forward again, then lift.

References

- Frontera, Walter R.; Slovik, David M.; Dawson, David Michael (2006), Exercise in Rehabilitation Medicine, Human Kinetics, 2006, p. 350, ISBN 978-0-7360-5541-3
- McMillian, Danny J.; Moore, Josef H.; Hatler, Brian S.; Taylor, Dean C. (2006-08-01). "Dynamic vs. static-stretching warm up: the effect on power and agility performance". Journal of Strength and Conditioning Research. 20 (3): 492–499. doi:10.1519/18205.1. ISSN 1064-8011. PMID 16937960
- Publishing, Harvard Health. "7 tips for a safe and successful strength-training program - Harvard Health". Harvard Health. Retrieved 2018-03-16
- Kingma, I.; Faber, G. S.; Suwarganda, E. K.; Bruijnen, T. B. M.; Peters, R. J. A.; Van Die??n, J. H. (2006). "Effect of a Stiff Lifting Belt on Spine Compression During Lifting". Spine. 31 (22): E833–E839. doi:10.1097/01.brs.0000240670.50834.77. PMID 17047531
- Rippetoe, Mark; Lon Kilgore (2005). "Squat". Starting Strength. The Aasgard Company. pp. 46–49. ISBN 0-9768054-0-5
- "MSNBC article on the U.S. Centers for Disease Control and Prevention report on the prevalence of strength training". Retrieved 2007-02-01

Chapter 6

Other Important Sports for Fitness

Regular exercise and sports maintain the overall health and wellness of the body and enhances physical fitness. Different sports help in maintaining physical fitness. Extensive importance is laid on sports, such as tennis, basketball, football, etc. in physical education, which have been thoroughly discussed in this chapter.

Tennis

Tennis, original name lawn tennis, game in which two opposing players (singles) or pairs of players (doubles) use tautly strung rackets to hit a ball of specified size, weight, and bounce over a net on a rectangular court. Points are awarded to a player or team whenever the opponent fails to correctly return the ball within the prescribed dimensions of the court. Organized tennis is played according to rules sanctioned by the International Tennis Federation (ITF), the world governing body of the sport.

While tennis can be enjoyed by players of practically any level of skill, top competition is a demanding test of both shot making and stamina, rich in stylistic and strategic variety. From its origins as a garden-party game for ladies in whalebone corsets and starched petticoats and men in long white flannels, it has evolved into a physical chess match in which players attack and defend, exploiting angles and technical weaknesses with strokes of widely diverse pace and spin. Tournaments offer tens of millions of dollars in prize money annually.

Types of Tennis Court

Clay

Clay courts are made of compressed shale, stone, or brick. While they are relatively easy and cheap to install, long-term maintenance can be quite expensive, particularly when compared to the costs of artificial tennis court surfaces. The water balance within the clay must be carefully monitored and adjusted, and the court must be rolled periodically to preserve its flatness.

In terms of play, clay courts are traditionally used in the French Open. These courts characteristically have a slower game and give balls a higher bounce. They tend to favor baseline players, as well. These courts are most popular in Europe and Latin America.

Grass

Tennis courts with grass surfaces are not as common today as they have been in the past due to the high maintenance costs of constant watering and mowing. They are also more impacted by weather conditions than clay or hard court surfaces are. Dirt is hard-packed and the grass must be trimmed very short. Grass is the fastest type of court because of its low bounce capacity. Players must get to the ball much more quickly than with clay or hard court. This means that players with stronger serve-and-volley skills will generally perform better. The grass court is the signature of Wimbledon.

Hard Courts

Hard courts can range from faster to slower speeds depending on the quantity and size of sand mixed into the paint coating. Hard courts tend to equalize the playing field in terms of athletic style. An acrylic hard court is used in the US Open and a synthetic for the Australian Open. While acrylic courts are more rigid and create a faster game, they can also be rough on the human body. To combat this, artificial tennis court surfaces were created to allow for similar usability and low maintenance, but also allow for greater shock absorption for players. These courts have been installed everywhere from the White House and the Sony Ericsson Open to high schools and tennis clubs around the world.

Carpet

Carpet courts are removable tennis court surfaces. These can be made from any of several materials, from artificial turf to hard rubber. In general, carpeted courts make for a fast game.

Types of Tennis Serve

The Flat Serve

For the Flat Serve, the server normally uses a Continental or an Eastern grip and swings directly through the ball, using no spin.

The key to a good Flat serve is power. Some professional players can hit them at over 150 mph.

The fastest serve ever recorded by a male player was 156 mph by Ivo Karlovic. The fastest serve ever recorded by a woman was 129 mph by Venus Williams.

The Slice Serve

For the slice serve, the server adopts a version of the Continental or Eastern backhand grip and brushes their racket across the right hand side of the ball (assuming the server is right handed, a left handed person brushes the left hand side of the ball), making the ball spin.

The sidespin makes the ball curve to the left and dip slightly, then bounce off the ground in a leftward direction (or rightward if the server is a lefty).

The slice serve can be used to go for an ace, to push the receiver off court and out of position, or to make the ball bounce up at the receiver's body.

The Kick Serve

The Kick Serve has been around since the end of the 19th Century. The ball is tossed up over the head and the racket brushes up and through it from roughly a 7 o'clock to 1 o'clock position.

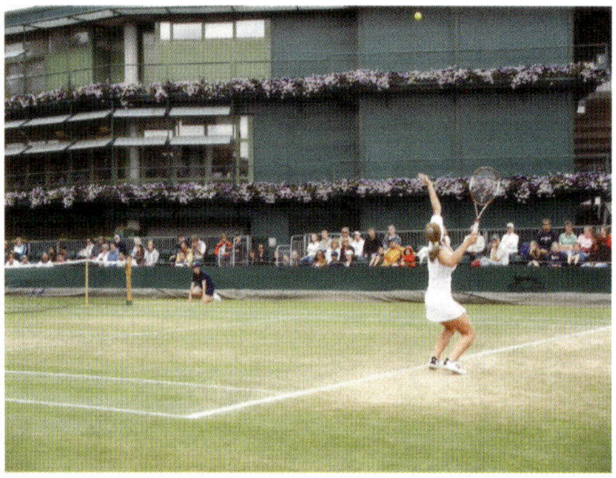

If done properly, the ball should arch over the net and then hit the ground with topspin and bounce up towards the receiver.

A variation of the Kick Serve is the American Twist, which is similar to the Kick, except that the spin is applied to the ball to make it bounce up and towards the left of the receiver, rather than straight at them.

The Underhanded Serve

Out of all the different types of tennis serve, serving underhand is the rarest. It is legitimate at all levels of the game, however, and can be employed at any time.

As it is so rare, it is often used to surprise an opponent.

One famous example of an underhand serve being used at the professional level occurred when Michael Chang famously beat Ivan Lendl in the 1989 French Open.

Benefits of Tennis

- Full body workout: Unlike some sports, playing tennis is a brilliant workout for the entire body. You use your lower body for all that running, stopping and starting, jumping and crouching. And the action of hitting the tennis ball, whether it's single or double-handed, means that your trunk does a lot of work as well, in particular your shoulders and upper back.
- Improved aerobic and anaerobic health: Tennis increases your oxygen intake while playing, increasing your heart rate and helping your blood deliver oxygen and nutrients to all your muscles. It also aids in the development of numerous capillaries and capillary beds within the muscles so that your muscles can have a greater blood supply and flow. This helps in your muscles perform at a higher level and fatigue at a slower rate. It also helps in maintaining anaerobic health, which allows the muscles to use oxygen in a better way and provide quick energy spurts for explosive power and quick, reactive movements.
- Burns calories and fat: Running, swinging, reaching, pivoting — tennis can be a real workout with the right opponent. It's a whole-body sport, and you can burn a lot of calories because

you're constantly on the move. In fact, for many people, playing tennis can actually burn more calories than other popular types of physical activity, including leisurely cycling, weight lifting, golfing, dancing or playing volleyball. As a result, playing tennis regularly has been shown to help reduce body fat. Singles tennis can burn between 400-600 calories an hour. That's not bad for a recreational sport that's both fun and can be played by just about anyone.

- Improves bone health: Playing tennis isn't good for your muscles alone; it has a positive impact on your bones as well. Exercising regularly can increase your peak bone mass and can slow the rate of bone mass loss over time. According to the National Institutes of Health (NIH), bone mass peaks around age 30 and begins to decline after that. You can maximize your bone mass prior to that age through exercise, and continuing to exercise after 30 can slow the rate of bone loss. The NIH names tennis as one of the weight-bearing activities well suited to building strong bones.
- Heart healthy: Tennis great Bjorn Borg accurately characterized a tennis match as "a thousand little sprints." The quick anaerobic movements the sport demands burns fat, increases your heart rate and promotes higher energy levels. A typical tennis match can last anywhere from one to two hours and at intervals that are optimal for improving cardiovascular health, which is essential for lowering your risk of heart disease, heart attack and stroke.
- Enhances flexibility, balance and coordination: Tennis requires the cooperation of the whole body. The feet maneuver you into the right position, the arms and hands position the racquet to make contact with the ball, and the torso and legs provide the power to send the ball flying over the net. All these factors come together every time you hit the ball, and each shot takes flexibility, coordination and balance. Flexibility is great because it can give you a wider range of motion, help prevent injuries and even reduce muscle strain.
- Boosts brain power: Tennis requires the brain to be creative, and it involves planning, tactical thinking, agility and the coordination of different parts of the body. So the more you play tennis, the better and stronger the neural connections related to those types of activities become, and the better you become at them. In addition to improving neural connections and developing new neurons, studies show that exercises that require a lot of thinking — such as tennis — can actually improve brain function in ways that aid memory, learning, social skills and behavior.
- Is great cross-training for other sports: Tennis involves quick-fire changes of direction at top speed as you race around the court to return serves and volleys. This requires 300 to 500 bursts of energy per match, according to researchers. And you'll run the equivalent of three to five miles. The effect? Playing tennis is a great way to speed up your sprinting and work on your endurance.
- Improves discipline and social skills: Tennis makes you more disciplined because the skills needed to master the game take patience, time and dedication. That's a lot of time spent practicing and focusing on getting better. Tennis helps you in achieving a better degree of socialization as you have to interact with different players.
- Boosts mood: Tennis players are more optimistic, have greater self-esteem and are less anxious, angry and depressed than people who play other sports or are sedentary, according to scientists in Connecticut.

Basketball

Basketball, game played between two teams of five players each on a rectangular court, usually indoors. Each team tries to score by tossing the ball through the opponent's goal, an elevated horizontal hoop and net called a basket.

Basic Positions in Basketball

1. Centre

The centre is generally the tallest player who is positioned near the basket as he must be able to get up as high as possible for rebounds. He is also required to be more physically domineering with more physical strength and overall athleticism.

Offensive -- The centre's goal is to get open for a pass and to shoot. They are required to block defenders, and to open other players up for driving to the basket for a goal. Centres are expected to get some offensive rebounds and put-backs.

The centre should be good at making quick jump shots, hook shots, and using the backboard on his shots.

Defensive -- On defense, the centre's main responsibility is to keep opponents from shooting by blocking shots and passes in the key area. They also are expected to get more rebounds because they're taller.

2. Power Forward

The power forwards are usually the next tallest players in the team, who are closest to the centre in physical attributes and playing style, but with more speed. A forward may play under the hoop or are expected to operate in the wings and corner areas.

They must be strong and comfortable with a lot of physical play and must be an effective rebounder and effective inside shooter like the centre. The power forward is also expected to shoot from further distances than the centre.

3. Small Forward

The small forward is usually the shorter of the two forwards on the team. However, the small forward must have enough height and ability to play inside, and on top of that, play like the centres and power forwards, but also be able to guard.

Small forwards are also the second or third best shooters from distance of the five positions as they also play defensive roles.

4. Shooting Guard

The shooting guard is potentially the shortest player in the team. However, he has to be good at dribbling fast, passing and having court vision by seeing the court. He is responsible for bringing the ball down the court and setting up offensive plays.

The shooting guard is also the player who takes the most shots. He needs to be an accurate shooter from three-point range.

The shooting guard is potentially the shortest player in the team. However, he has to be good at dribbling fast, passing and having court vision by seeing the court. He is responsible for bringing the ball down the court and setting up offensive plays. In terms of height, shooting guards are taller than point guards.

5. Point Guard

The point guard needs to be the best ball handler, dribbler and passer as he handles the ball the most out of all the players on the team. He needs to bring the ball down the court and initiate offensive plays.

Point guards can also be the shortest player on the team as they use their intelligence and court vision to coordinate all his teammates on offense.

Point guards need to have a good long distance shooting, though it's not quite as crucial as for shooting guards. However, some point guards take as many shots as shooting guards.

Basketball Rules

The rules of basketball can vary slightly depending on the level of play or where the game is played. These rule differences, however, are usually just variations on the basic game of basketball and the majority of the rules discussed below can be applied to most any game of basketball played.

The winner of a basketball game is the team with the most points. You get points by throwing the basketball through the opponent's hoop or basket. In regular play a basket made from within the three point line is worth 2 points and a basket shot from outside the three point line is worth three points. When shooting a free throw, each free throw is worth 1 point.

Rules for the Offense

The basketball team on offense is the team with the basketball. When a player has the basketball there are certain rules they must follow:

1) The player must bounce, or dribble, the ball with one hand while moving both feet. If, at any time, both hands touch the ball or the player stops dribbling, the player must only move one foot. The foot that is stationary is called the pivot foot.

2) The basketball player can only take one turn at dribbling. In other words, once a player has stopped dribbling they cannot start another dribble. A player who starts dribbling again is called for a double-dribbling violation and looses the basketball to the other team. A player can only start another dribble after another player from either team touches or gains control of the basketball. This is usually after a shot or pass.

3) The ball must stay in bounds. If the offensive team looses the ball out of bounds the other team gets control of the basketball.

4) The players hand must be on top of the ball while dribbling. If they touch the bottom of the basketball while dribbling and continue to dribble this is called carrying the ball and the player will lose the ball to the other team.

5) Once the offensive team crosses half court, they may not go back into the backcourt. This is called a backcourt violation. If the defensive team knocks the ball into the backcourt, then the offensive team can recover the ball legally.

Defensive Rules

The team on defense is the team without the basketball.

1) The main rule for the defensive player is not to foul. A foul is described as gaining an unfair advantage through physical contact. There is some interpretation that has to be made by the referee, but, in general, the defensive player may not touch the offensive player in a way that causes the offensive player to lose the ball or miss a shot.

Rules for Everyone

1) Although the foul rule is described above as a defensive rule, it applies exactly the same to all players on the court including offensive players.

2) Basketball players cannot kick the ball or hit it with their fist.

3) No player can touch the basketball while it is traveling downward towards the basket or if it is on the rim. This is called goaltending.

Every player on the court is subject to the same rules regardless of the position they play. The positions in basketball are just for team basketball strategy and there are no positions in the rules.

Three Types of Basketballs

- *Leather* – these basketballs are made from 100% genuine leather cover. When a leather ball is new, it may feel somewhat hard to feel, but with a bit of wear, it becomes soft having an appealing broken-in feel. Leather basketballs are strictly for indoor hardwood court only because the feel of the leather will roughen when used on concrete surfaces. Leather basketballs are also the most expensive of the three types of basketballs.

- *Composite / Synthetic Leather* – these basketballs are covered with artificial or synthetic leather material that has the feel of leather, as it has been designed that way, but much cheaper to produce and manufacture. Since it is synthetic, the material has a uniform feel which is why it does not need to be broken-in as it already has that soft feel even when new.

- *Rubber* – these basketballs are lined with rubber covering and are ideal for concrete surfaces. Rubber basketballs are perfect for beginners, especially since they are the cheapest to produce.

Benefits of Basketball

- Burns calories: Running, jumping and quick lateral movements done in basketball provide a significant amount of aerobic exercise and can burn a great deal of calories. For each hour of competitive basketball, a 165-pound person can expect to burn around 600 calories, while a 250-pound person can burn up to 900 calories.
- Great for cardiovascular health: Basketball can help you develop cardiovascular endurance, depending on how many times play stops. Keep moving and you'll keep your heart rate up. Building endurance can help keep your heart healthy, reducing the risk of heart disease and stroke later in life.
- Develops concentration and self-discipline: Like every other sport, basketball has rules to follow, and breaking them can result in penalties not just for you, but for your team. Practicing self-discipline helps one become more competitive yet fair and clean in their game and focused in succeeding.
- Builds bone strength: Jumping and other physical demands of basketball help develop and improve bone health. The stronger your bones, the less likely they are to break. Weight-bearing physical activity causes new bone tissue to form, making bones stronger. Bones and muscles both become stronger when muscles push and tug against bones during physical activity.
- Better motor skills and coordination: Free-throw shooting and jump-shooting are particularly helpful for training hand-eye coordination. Rebounding missed shots is another skill that requires a great degree of full-body coordination. The third basic basketball skill, dribbling, requires a finer degree of coordination. When first learning basketball, dribbling trains the hand-eye coordination; once that skilled is mastered, a player will no longer look at the ball while dribbling and the skill will become a pure motor coordination task.
- Strength training: Basketball provides an excellent full-body workout and can help develop useful, lean muscle. In this physically intensive contact sport, basketball players are highly reliant on effective body positioning and the ability to maintain that position when an opponent is pushing against him. Playing good defensive basketball can develop your deltoids, traps, neck, lower back and core muscles. Strong legs aid in shooting and running, while the finer movements such as dribbling and shooting are good for strengthening your arms, wrist flexors and hand muscles.
- Improves spatial awareness: Spatial awareness is knowing where your body is in space and time. Ever wonder why a cat always lands on its feet? Body awareness. It helps keep you in balance.
- Mental development: Basketball requires a wide range of physical skills, but it is also a fast-paced mental game. Research on the mental aspects of basketball has revealed that players must develop a great deal of attention to quickly and accurately process what's happening on the court and make effective decisions with the ball and on defense. During a fast-paced game, you must train yourself to constantly observe your teammates and opponents and evaluate what course of action to take in response to

their actions. This can translate to helping you make quick decisions on the job and in other real-life situations.

- o Reduces stress and boosts the immune system: Decreasing your stress will help you focus and have more energy to complete tasks. Playing basketball and other sports helps reduce stress and gives players the opportunity to socialize. People who are social are less likely to have depression, and also tend to have a stronger immune system.
- o Enhances confidence: Basketball truly improves anyone's confidence. Making good shots and being a part of a good team can increase your self-esteem and help gain more confidence. A confident person has more faith in his or her skills and can face life with a better disposition.

Football

Football, also called association football or soccer, game in which two teams of 11 players, using any part of their bodies except their hands and arms, try to maneuver the ball into the opposing team's goal. Only the goalkeeper is permitted to handle the ball and may do so only within the penalty area surrounding the goal. The team that scores more goals wins.

Football is the world's most popular ball game in numbers of participants and spectators. Simple in its principal rules and essential equipment, the sport can be played almost anywhere, from official football playing fields (pitches) to gymnasiums, streets, school playgrounds, parks, or beaches. Football's governing body, the Fédération Internationale de Football Association (FIFA), estimated that at the turn of the 21st century there were approximately 250 million football players and over 1.3 billion people "interested" in football; in 2010 a combined television audience of more than 26 billion watched football's premier tournament, the quadrennial month-long World Cup finals.

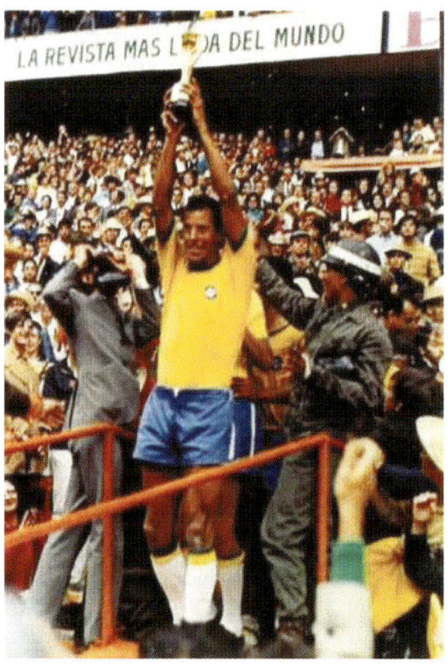

Captain Carlos Alberto Torres holding the Jules Rimet trophy at the World Cup.

Shape and Size

Unlike the balls used in most sports, a football is not spherical in shape, so there is more of an unpredictability in the way it bounces. When thrown, ideally the ball leaves the hand spinning in a spiral motion, which keeps the flight of the ball more aerodynamic.

There are different sizes of footballs, with smaller versions available for youth play. At the NFL level, the ball measures from 20 3/4 to 21 1/4 inches around its middle, 28 to 28 1/2 inches around its ends and 11 to 11 1/4 inches from tip to tip.

Inflation Level

The football also weighs between 14 and 15 ounces and is inflated to between 12 1/2 and 13 1/2 pounds per square inch. The inflation level of footballs is important. During the 2014-2015 NFL playoffs, most of the balls used in the first half of a game between the New England Patriots and the Indianapolis Colts were found to be about 2 pounds under the minimum required inflation level. A complaint from the Colts prompted the referees to test inflation levels and investigate.

The Patriots, who were hosting the game, received some blame for the underinflation. The issue even sparked a controversy called "Deflategate," and quarterback Tom Brady eventually received a four-game suspension because the NFL found that Brady may have known about the underinflation.

Benefits of Football

Cardiovascular and Health Benefits

Football involves running, sprinting and drills that require generous energy expenditure and engage the cardiovascular system. Regularly participating in aerobic exercise such as football offers benefits such as increased longevity, as well as reduced susceptibility to heart disease, osteoporosis, diabetes and other chronic diseases. It can also foster weight loss and weight management; a 155-pound person burns nearly 600 calories per hour playing football. Football players, particularly those who are overweight, may lose 15 to 20 pounds in a single season.

Fitness Skills

Football helps develop numerous types of fitness skills including speed, agility and power. Players may lose body fat, gain lean muscle and increase the likelihood of maintaining healthy habits throughout life. Football players will develop muscle strength through conditioning exercises and explosive power through tackling and defensive moves. Other advantageous elements of football include increased muscular endurance, as well as improved flexibly and mobility.

Psychological and Social Benefits

Abiding by the rules of the game and adhering to the coach's instruction teaches players discipline and emotional temperance. The competitive aspect of the game helps the players learn how to deal with disappointment, develop resilience, practice good sportsmanship and learn how to grow from constructive criticism. Football can also instill confidence and self-esteem, and help players overcome shyness, Cisar explains. The fast-paced nature of the game requires players to harness a great deal of concentration, adaptability and quick thinking. Football can also help ward off depression, as well as help players develop positive social circles and role models.

Permissions

All chapters in this book are published with permission under the Creative Commons Attribution Share Alike License or equivalent. Every chapter published in this book has been scrutinized by our experts. Their significance has been extensively debated. The topics covered herein carry significant information for a comprehensive understanding. They may even be implemented as practical applications or may be referred to as a beginning point for further studies.

We would like to thank the editorial team for lending their expertise to make the book truly unique. They have played a crucial role in the development of this book. Without their invaluable contributions this book wouldn't have been possible. They have made vital efforts to compile up to date information on the varied aspects of this subject to make this book a valuable addition to the collection of many professionals and students.

This book was conceptualized with the vision of imparting up-to-date and integrated information in this field. To ensure the same, a matchless editorial board was set up. Every individual on the board went through rigorous rounds of assessment to prove their worth. After which they invested a large part of their time researching and compiling the most relevant data for our readers.

The editorial board has been involved in producing this book since its inception. They have spent rigorous hours researching and exploring the diverse topics which have resulted in the successful publishing of this book. They have passed on their knowledge of decades through this book. To expedite this challenging task, the publisher supported the team at every step. A small team of assistant editors was also appointed to further simplify the editing procedure and attain best results for the readers.

Apart from the editorial board, the designing team has also invested a significant amount of their time in understanding the subject and creating the most relevant covers. They scrutinized every image to scout for the most suitable representation of the subject and create an appropriate cover for the book.

The publishing team has been an ardent support to the editorial, designing and production team. Their endless efforts to recruit the best for this project, has resulted in the accomplishment of this book. They are a veteran in the field of academics and their pool of knowledge is as vast as their experience in printing. Their expertise and guidance has proved useful at every step. Their uncompromising quality standards have made this book an exceptional effort. Their encouragement from time to time has been an inspiration for everyone.

The publisher and the editorial board hope that this book will prove to be a valuable piece of knowledge for students, practitioners and scholars across the globe.

Index